AF760917

MICROBIOLOGICAL RISK ASSESSMENT SERIES

8

# Risk assessment of *Vibrio vulnificus* in raw oysters

INTERPRETATIVE SUMMARY
AND TECHNICAL REPORT

WORLD HEALTH ORGANIZATION

FOOD AND AGRICULTURE ORGANIZATION OF THE UNITED NATIONS

2005

WHO Library Cataloguing-in-Publication Data

Risk assessment of *Vibrio vulnificus* in raw oysters: interpretative summary and technical report.

Published jointly with the Food and Agriculture Organization of the United Nations (FAO).

(Microbiological risk assessment series No. 8)
1. *Vibrio vulnificus* – growth & development 2. *Vibrio vulnificus* – pathogenicity 3. Oysters – microbiology 4. Oysters – pathogenicity. 5. Risk assessment 6. Food contamination I. Food and Agriculture Organization of the United Nations II. World Health Organization III. Title IV. Series.

ISBN 92 4 156310 9 (WHO) (NLM classification: QW 141)
ISBN 92 5 105423 1 (FAO)
ISSN 1726-5274

# CONTENTS

# ACKNOWLEDGEMENTS

The Food and Agriculture Organization of the United Nations and the World Health Organization would like to express their appreciation to all those who contributed to the preparation of this report. Special appreciation is extended to the risk assessment drafting group on *Vibrio* spp. in seafood, and in particular the core group on risk assessment of *Vibrio vulnificus* in raw oysters, for the time and effort that they freely dedicated to the elaboration of this assessment. Many people provided their time and expertise by reviewing the report and providing their comments, additional data and other relevant information. Both the risk assessment drafting group and the reviewers are listed in the following pages.

Appreciation is also extended to all those who responded to the calls for data that were issued by FAO and WHO and brought to our attention data not readily available in the mainstream literature and official documentation.

The risk assessment work was coordinated by the Secretariat of the Joint FAO/WHO Expert Meetings on Microbiological Risk Assessment (JEMRA). This included Sarah Cahill, Maria de Lourdes Costarrica and Jean-Louis Jouve (2001-2004) in FAO, and Peter Karim Ben Embarek, Jocelyne Rocourt (2001- 2004), Hajime Toyofuku (1999-2004) and Jørgen Schlundt in WHO. During the development of the risk assessment, additional support and feedback were provided by Lahsen Ababouch, Henri Loreal and Hector Lupin, Fishery Industries Division in FAO, and Jeronimas Maskeliunas, Codex Secretariat. Sarah Cahill coordinated the finalisation and publication of the report. Thorgeir Lawrence was responsible for editing the report for language and preparation for printing.

The preparatory work and the publication of this report was supported and funded by the FAO Food Quality and Standards Service, the FAO Fishery Industries Division and the WHO Department of Food Safety, Zoonoses and Foodborne Disease.

.

# RISK ASSESSMENT DRAFTING GROUP

**John Bowers***

Center for Food Safety and Applied Nutrition, United States Food and Drug Administration, United States of America

**Anders Dalsgaard**

Department of Veterinary Microbiology, The Royal Veterinary and Agricultural University, Denmark

**Angelo DePaola***

Office of Seafood, Center for Food Safety and Applied Nutrition, United States Food and Drug Administration, United States of America

**I. Karunasagar**

Department of Fishery Microbiology, University of Agricultural Sciences College of Fisheries, India

**Thomas McMeekin**

Centre for Food Safety and Quality, University of Tasmania, Australia

**Mitsuaki Nishibuchi**

Center for Southeast Asian Studies, Kyoto University, Japan

**Ken Osaka**

National Institute of Infectious Diseases, Ministry of Health, Labour and Welfare, Japan

**John Sumner**

M&S Food Consultants Pty. Ltd., Australia

**Mark Walderhaug**

Center for Food Safety and Applied Nutrition, United States Food and Drug Administration, United States of America

---

* Members of core group on risk assessment of *Vibrio vulnificus* in raw oysters

# REVIEWERS

## Participants in expert consultations

| | |
|---|---|
| **Awa Kane Aïdara** | Institut Pasteur de Dakar, Laboratoire de Bactériologie Expérimentale, Senegal. |
| **Nourredine Bouchriti** | Department d'Hygiéne et d'Industrie des Denrées Alimentaires d'Origine Animale, Institut Agronomique et Vétérinaire Hassan II, Morocco. |
| **Jean-Michel Fournier** | Centre National de Référence des Vibrions et du Choléra, Institut Pasteur, France. |
| **Ron Lee** | Centre for Environment, Fisheries and Aquaculture Science, Weymouth Laboratory, United Kingdom. |
| **Carlos Lima dos Santos** | Private Consultant, Brazil. |
| **Dorothy-Jean McCoubrey** | Ministry of Agriculture and Forestry, New Zealand. |
| **Marianne Miliotis** | Center for Food Safety and Applied Nutrition, United States Food and Drug Administration, United States of America. |
| **Noel Murray** | Biosecurity Authority, Ministry of Agriculture and Forestry, New Zealand. |
| **Pensri Rodma** | Department of Medical Science, Ministry of Public Health, Thailand. |
| **Mark Tamplin** | Eastern Regional Research Center – North Atlantic Area, United States Department of Agriculture, United States of America. |
| **Paul Vanderlinde** | Food Science Australia, Australia |
| **Shigeki Yamamoto** | National Institute of Infectious Diseases, Ministry of Health, Labour and Welfare, Japan. |

## Peer reviewers

| | |
|---|---|
| **Kimitaka Sagawa** | Department of Laboratory Medicine, Kurume University School of Medicine, Japan. |
| **Marleen M. Wekell** | Office of Research, Center for Veterinary Medicine, United States of America. |

| | |
|---|---|
| **James D. Oliver** | Department of Biology, University of North Carolina, United States of America. |
| **Mark Powell** | United States Department of Agriculture, United States of America. |
| **Lee-Ann Jaykus** | Departments of Food Science and Microbiology, North Carolina State University, United States of America. |
| **Rachel Rangdale** | The Centre for Environment, Fisheries and Aquaculture Science, Weymouth Laboratory, United Kingdom. |
| **Joon Haeng Rhee** | National Research Laboratory of Molecular Microbial Pathogenesis and Department of Microbiology, Chonnam National University Medical School, Republic of Korea. |
| **John Painter** | Centers for Disease Control, Foodborne and Diarrheal Diseases Branch, United States of America. |
| **Dan Herman** and **Robert Collette** | National Fisheries Institute, United States of America. |

# FOREWORD

The Members of the Food and Agriculture Organization of the United Nations (FAO) and of the World Health Organization (WHO) have expressed concern regarding the level of safety of food both at national and international levels. Increasing foodborne disease incidence over the last decades seems, in many countries, to be related to an increase in disease caused by microorganisms in food. This concern has been voiced in meetings of the Governing Bodies of both Organizations and in the Codex Alimentarius Commission. It is not easy to decide whether the suggested increase is real or an artefact of changes in other areas, such as improved disease surveillance or better detection methods for microorganisms in foods. However, the important issue is whether new tools or revised and improved actions can contribute to our ability to lower the disease burden and provide safer food. Fortunately new tools, which can facilitate actions, seem to be on their way.

Over the past decade, Risk Analysis – a process consisting of risk assessment, risk management and risk communication – has emerged as a structured model for improving our food control systems with the objectives of producing safer food, reducing the numbers of foodborne illnesses and facilitating domestic and international trade in food. Furthermore, we are moving towards a more holistic approach to food safety, where the entire food chain needs to be considered in efforts to produce safer food.

As with any model, tools are needed for the implementation of the risk analysis paradigm. Risk assessment is the science-based component of risk analysis. Science today provides us with in-depth information on life in the world we live in. It has allowed us to accumulate a wealth of knowledge on microscopic organisms, their growth, survival and death, even their genetic make-up. It has given us an understanding of food production, processing and preservation, and of the link between the microscopic and the macroscopic world and how we can benefit from as well as suffer from these microorganisms. Risk assessment provides us with a framework for organizing all this data and information and to better understand the interaction between microorganisms, foods and human illness. It provides us with the ability to estimate the risk to human health from specific microorganisms in foods and gives us a tool with which we can compare and evaluate different scenarios, as well as to identify the types of data necessary for estimating and optimizing mitigating interventions.

Microbiological risk assessment can be considered as a tool that can be used in the management of the risks posed by foodborne pathogens and in the elaboration of standards for food in international trade. However, undertaking a microbiological risk assessment (MRA), particularly quantitative MRA, is recognized as a resource-intensive task requiring a multidisciplinary approach. Yet foodborne illness is among the most widespread public health problems, creating social and economic burdens as well as human suffering, making it a concern that all countries need to address. As risk assessment can also be used to justify the introduction of more stringent standards for imported foods, a knowledge of MRA is important for trade purposes, and there is a need to provide countries with the tools for understanding and, if possible, undertaking MRA. This need, combined with that of the Codex Alimentarius for risk-based scientific advice, led FAO and WHO to undertake a programme of activities on MRA at the international level.

The Food Quality and Standards Service, FAO, and the Department of Food Safety, Zoonoses and Foodborne Disease, WHO, are the lead units responsible for this initiative. The two groups have worked together to develop the area of MRA at the international level for application at both the national and international levels. This work has been greatly facilitated by the contribution of people from around the world with expertise in microbiology, mathematical modelling, epidemiology and food technology to name but a few.

This Microbiological Risk Assessment series provides a range of data and information to those who need to understand or undertake MRA. It comprises risk assessments of particular pathogen-commodity combinations, interpretative summaries of the risk assessments, guidelines for undertaking and using risk assessment, and reports addressing other pertinent aspects of MRA.

We hope that this series will provide a greater insight into MRA, how it is undertaken and how it can be used. We strongly believe that this is an area that should be developed in the international sphere, and have already from the present work clear indications that an international approach and early agreement in this area will strengthen the future potential for use of this tool in all parts of the world, as well as in international standard setting. We would welcome comments and feedback on any of the documents within this series so that we can endeavour to provide Member countries, Codex Alimentarius and other users of this material with the information they need to use risk-based tools, with the ultimate objective of ensuring that safe food is available for all consumers.

***Ezzeddine Boutrif***

Food Quality and Standards Service
FAO

***Jørgen Schlundt***

Department of Food Safety, Zoonoses and
Foodborne Disease, WHO

# BACKGROUND

In response to a request from Codex for scientific advice, FAO and WHO, in 2001, established a risk assessment drafting group and convened an expert consultation to take the first steps in developing a risk assessment on *Vibrio* spp. in seafood products that would have the most impact on public health and/or international trade. The expert consultation concluded that three species, *Vibrio parahaemolyticus*, *Vibrio vulnificus*, and choleragenic *Vibrio cholerae* were the species responsible for most cases of human illness caused by vibrios, and several seafood vehicles associated with these illnesses were identified. Work was thus undertaken on the following pathogen-product combinations:

- *V. parahaemolyticus* in raw oysters harvested and consumed in Japan, New Zealand, Australia, Canada and the United States of America.
- *V. parahaemolyticus* in finfish consumed raw.
- *V. parahaemolyticus* in bloody clams harvested and consumed in Thailand.
- *V. vulnificus* in raw oysters harvested and consumed in the United States of America.
- Choleragenic *V. cholerae* O1 and O139 in warm-water shrimp in international trade.

These five individual risk assessments illustrate how different approaches were used to reflect the national capacity to generate data, including health statistics and data on the pathogen and the commodity of concern. The assessments considered information on *Vibrio* spp. in seafood that was generated and available at regional and national levels and this information formed the substantive basis from which the risk assessments were developed.

The current document describes the risk assessment of *V. vulnificus* in raw oysters. When this work began, a draft risk assessment model had been developed in the United States of America to assess the public health risk associated with *V. parahaemolyticus* in raw oysters. The above-mentioned FAO/WHO *V. parahaemolyticus* risk assessment in raw oysters looked at how to adapt the model developed in the USA to the situation in other countries. The purpose of this risk assessment was to investigate further the utility of the United States draft *V. parahaemolyticus* model, which was published in 2001[1], together with the additional work undertaken by FAO and WHO on the risk assessment of *V. parahaemolyticus*, and determine if it could be adapted to a different pathogen, *V. vulnificus*. The current risk assessment was developed in the same raw oyster vehicle and also, for reasons of data availability, for the same geographic region, thereby representing a very similar exposure scenario. This risk assessment was also undertaken because *V. vulnificus* illness has one of the highest mortality rates of any foodborne disease and has emerged as a food safety issue in a number of countries and regions including Europe, Japan, New Zealand, Republic of Korea and the USA.

---

[1] The final version of the United Stated Food and Drug Administrations Quantitative Risk Assessment on the Public Health Impact of Pathogenic *Vibrio parahaemolyticus* In Raw Oysters was released on 20th July 2005. This current work does not take into account any changes that were made to the original draft model (2001) and which were included in this just published version of the risk assessment.

# ABBREVIATIONS

| | |
|---|---|
| AIDS | Acquired Immune Deficiency Syndrome |
| CAC | Codex Alimentarius Commission |
| CCFH | Codex Committee on Food Hygiene |
| CDC | Centers for Disease Control (USA) |
| COVISS | Cholera and other Vibrios Surveillance System |
| FAO | Food and Agriculture Organization of the United Nations |
| FAO/WHO-VPRA | Joint FAO/WHO Risk Assessment of *V. parahaemolyticus* in Raw Oysters |
| FDA | Food and Drug Administration (USA) |
| FDA-VPRA | U.S. FDA Draft Risk Assessment on the Public Health Impacts of *V. parahaemolyticus* in Raw Molluscan Shellfish |
| g | gram |
| GCSL | FDA Gulf Coast Seafood Laboratory, Dauphin Island (USA) |
| ICP | Interim Control Plan for *Vibrio parahaemolyticus* |
| ISSC | Interstate Shellfish Sanitation Conference (USA) |
| Kg | Kilogram |
| LOD | Limit of detection |
| MLE | Maximum Likelihood Estimate |
| MPN | Most Probable Number |
| NBDC | National Buoy Data Center (USA) |
| NERRS | National Estuarine Research Reserve System (USA) |
| NOAA | National Oceanic and Atmospheric Administration (USA) |
| NSSP | National Shellfish Sanitation Program (USA) |
| PCR | Polymerase Chain Reaction |
| ppt | parts per thousand |
| RAPD | Random Amplification of Polymorphic DNA |
| USDA | United States Department of Agriculture |
| VBNC | Viable but non-culturable |
| VPRA | *Vibrio parahaemolyticus* Risk Assessment |
| Vv | *Vibrio vulnificus* |
| WHO | World Health Organization |

# INTERPRETATIVE SUMMARY

# INTRODUCTION

This risk assessment was undertaken as one of five pathogen-commodity combinations addressed in the FAO/WHO risk assessment work on *Vibrio* spp. in seafood. Within that framework *Vibrio vulnificus* was identified as one of the three *Vibrio* spp. responsible for most cases of human illness caused by vibrios, where seafood was the vehicle of transmission. There have been at least two previous risk assessments for *Vibrio vulnificus*. McCoubrey (1996) reported on the risk of *V. vulnificus* infection following consumption of raw commercially harvested North Island oysters from New Zealand in 1996. The European Commission's Scientific Committee on Veterinary Measures relating to Public Health has prepared a document on *V. vulnificus* and *Vibrio parahaemolyticus* in raw and undercooked seafood (Scientific Committee on Veterinary Measures relating to Public Health, 2001). However, neither of these risk assessments was quantitative.

In considering approaches to undertake a risk assessment on this pathogen in seafood, with limited available resources, it was decided to extend the *V. parahaemolyticus* models described in the United States FDA "Draft Risk Assessment on the Public Health Impacts of *V. parahaemolyticus* in Raw Molluscan Shellfish" ("FDA-VPRA") (FDA, 2001) and the Joint FAO/WHO Risk Assessment of *V. parahaemolyticus* in raw oysters ("FAO/WHO-VPRA") (FAO/WHO, in press) to *V. vulnificus*. The general approach and many of the parameters used in the current *V. vulnificus* risk assessment are the same as those used in the draft FDA-VPRA and FAO/WHO-VPRA.

## Objective and scope

The first objective of this risk assessment was to determine the usefulness of adapting the FDA-VPRA and FAO/WHO-VPRA models to assess the risk from *V. vulnificus* septicaemia associated with the consumption of raw oysters. Secondly, the risk assessment aimed to identify the most appropriate data, as well as gaps in the available dataset, for modelling purposes. In addition to estimating the risk of *V. vulnificus* septicaemia associated with the consumption of raw oysters, the risk assessment model was also developed with the objective of evaluating targeted mitigation levels aimed at reducing the risk of *V. vulnificus* septicaemia. For reasons of data availability, the risk assessment was limited to consideration of primary septicaemia cases associated with consumption of raw oysters from the Gulf Coast of the United States of America (USA).

# HAZARD IDENTIFICATION

*V. vulnificus* naturally inhabits warm estuarine environments and can infect humans via wound exposure or seafood consumption. These infections are rare and generally limited to individuals with pre-existing chronic illnesses or the immunocompromised. However, *V. vulnificus* can invade through the intestinal barrier into the bloodstream causing primary septicaemia. As a result, it has the highest case/fatality rate (approx. 50%) among foodborne pathogens. While *V. vulnificus* has been found in a variety of seafood's worldwide and illnesses have been reported in a number of countries, its epidemiology, ecology and distribution in seafood's have been most extensively investigated in the USA. Each year, 30 to 40 oyster-associated primary septicaemia cases are reported in the USA and nearly all of these are associated with the consumption of raw oysters harvested from the Gulf Coast in the south of that country.

## EXPOSURE ASSESSMENT

A schematic diagram of the *V. vulnificus* risk assessment model is shown in Figure 1. Modelling exposure to *V. vulnificus* followed the same approach and used many of the same assumptions as used for the FAO/WHO-VPRA and the FDA-VPRA. The model inputs, data sources and assumptions are summarized in Table 1.

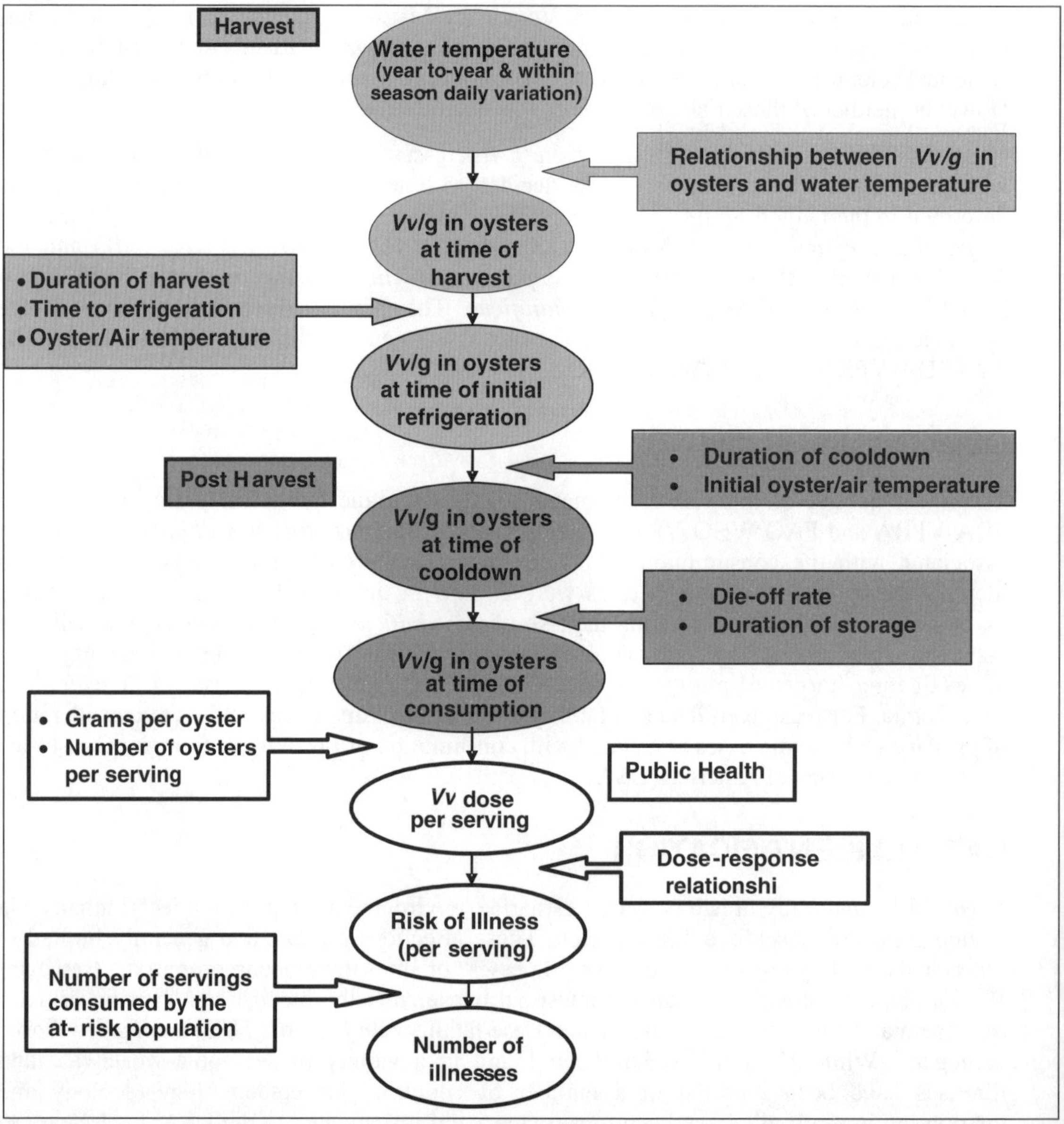


**Figure 1.** *V. vulnificus* (*Vv*) conceptual risk assessment model showing integration of all modules.

**Table 1**. Model inputs, data sources and assumptions for the proposed *V. vulnificus* risk assessment

| Model Inputs | Data Source | Assumptions |
|---|---|---|
| Water temperature | FAO/WHO-VPRA/FDA-VPRA; NOAA buoy data (NOAA, 1999); and NERRS (NERRS, 2001) | Buoy and other fixed site data are representative of growing areas. |
| Total *V. vulnificus* numbers at harvest | Weekly oyster samples from 4 Gulf States 1994–1995 (Motes et al., 1998; Tamplin, 1994) | Data relevant for other years. |
| Pathogenic *V. vulnificus* numbers at harvest | Weekly oyster samples from 4 Gulf States 1994–1995 (Motes et al., 1998; Tamplin, 1994) | All *V. vulnificus* strains are equally virulent. Data from Jackson, Murphree and Tamplin (1997) and two recent studies (Nilsson et al., 2003; DePaola et al., 2003) suggest opposing view on this subject, but neither addresses seasonal or regional differences in virulence. |
| Air temperature | FAO/WHO-VPRA/FDA-VPRA; NOAA buoy data (NOAA, 1999) | Temperature of oyster meat equilibrates rapidly to that of air. |
| Time harvest vessel in water | FAO/WHO-VPRA/FDA-VPRA; Dealer survey (Cook, 1997b) | Harvest practices have not changed since 1996. |
| Time to first refrigeration | FAO/WHO-VPRA/FDA-VPRA; Dealer survey (Cook, 1997b) | Oysters are harvested at a constant rate throughout the harvest period. |
| *V. vulnificus* growth rate | Natural populations in oysters at ambient temperature (Cook, 1997a). Data lacking at lower temperature | *V. vulnificus* grows at similar temperature-specific rates in Gulf oysters from April to October. |
| *V. vulnificus*/g at first refrigeration | Dealer survey of Gulf oysters 1995–1996 (Cook, 1997b) | Dealer practices in 1996 are typical of current practices. |
| Cool down time | FAO/WHO-VPRA/FDA-VPRA; no data | Rectangular (uniform) distribution between 1 and 10 h. |
| *V. vulnificus*/g at cool down | Dealer survey of Gulf oysters 1995–1996 (Cook, 1997b) | Dealer practices in 1996 are typical of current practices. |
| *V. vulnificus* survival | Natural populations in oysters stored at 3°C for 14-17 d (Cook et al., 2002) | *V. vulnificus* die off at 3°C similar to that at other temperatures between 0-13°C. |
| Pathogenic *V. vulnificus*/g at consumption | Retail study of USA oysters 1998–1999 (Cook et al., 2002) | Data are relevant for other years. (The autumn of 1998 was extremely warm and *V. vulnificus* levels were considerably higher than levels predicted for typical autumn temperatures). |
| Percentage of population susceptible | Prevalence of liver disease, immune disorder, etc., in the USA (Klontz, 1997; Desenclos et al., 1991; Shapiro et al., 1998; Hlady, 1997) | All predisposing conditions have been identified and risk of infection is homogeneous with respect to these conditions. There is no risk of illness (septicaemia) to individuals without the identified disease conditions. |
| Percentage of oysters consumed raw | 50% oysters consumed raw; FAO/WHO-VPRA | Susceptible individuals consume raw oysters at the same rate as the total population. |
| No. of oysters per serving | FAO/WHO-VPRA/FDA-VPRA | Consumption behaviour has not changed appreciably in recent years. |
| Weight per oyster | Retail study of USA oysters 1998–1999 (Cook et al., 2002) | None. |
| Risk of illness | Relationship between monthly exposure and illness within defined (Gulf States) population (Cook et al., 2002; M. Glatzer, personal communication, 2001; NMFS, 1998) | Consumption of raw oysters among the susceptible population does not vary from month to month. (If the percentage of raw oysters consumed was greater in cooler months, the effect of the assumption would be to over-predict the risk at lower *V. vulnificus* levels).<br>Reporting of *V. vulnificus* septicaemia cases related to oyster consumption does not vary from month to month. |
| Number of illnesses | Risk of illness (from above) multiplied by number of servings | Same as above for risk of illness. |

The assumption that all strains are equally virulent is based primarily on animal models (DePaola et al., 2003) that may not be valid for humans, as is suggested by other studies. Those of Jackson, Murphree and Tamplin (1997) and Nilsson et al. (2003) indicate that only a few strains of the diverse populations of *V. vulnificus* found in oysters are associated with human disease. However, there is no definitive test available to measure virulence and no data available to determine their seasonal and regional distribution or their ability to grow and survive under typical industry practices and proposed interventions. Thus, in the absence of definitive information to the contrary, it was assumed that all strains are equally virulent.

Like *V. parahaemolyticus*, *V. vulnificus* numbers at harvest are determined primarily by water temperature and salinity. Other factors may also contribute to *V. vulnificus* numbers but only temperature and salinity have been quantified (Motes et al., 1998; Tamplin, 1994). The numbers of *V. vulnificus* at consumption are influenced by the ambient air temperatures at harvest; the time from harvest until the oysters are placed under refrigeration; the time it takes the oysters to cool once under refrigeration; and the length of refrigeration time until consumption. The growth model used in the present assessment is the three-phase linear growth model advocated for microbial risk assessment by Buchanan, Whiting and Damert (1997).

Two data sets were identified for estimating total *V. vulnificus* numbers relative to the water temperature at harvest. Analyses of these data sets separately and combined pointed to substantial differences, which indicated that it was not appropriate to combine them (simplistically) into a single (pooled) data set. The sensitivity of the exposure assessment to the apparent differences between these data sets was evaluated by conducting alternative assessments based on each data set separately as well as combined (or pooled). The results of these analyses were then compared with available data on the density of *V. vulnificus* in oysters at retail (Cook et al., 2002) for validation. This comparative validation approach suggested that the estimates based on the Motes et al. (1998) dataset were a more appropriate basis for model predictions.

Overall, the model simulation results suggest that *V. vulnificus* numbers increase post-harvest an average of 0.90 $\log_{10}$ MPN per gram during the summer harvest season and decrease an average of 0.2 $\log_{10}$ MPN per gram during the winter harvest season. Mean densities of 57 000 and 80 organisms per gram were obtained for the summer and winter harvest seasons, respectively. Given an average serving size of 196 g of oyster meat (Cook et al., 2002; A. DePaola, personal communication, 2002), these mean densities correspond to average ingested doses of $1.1 \times 10^7$ and $1.6 \times 10^4$ respectively.

## HAZARD CHARACTERIZATION

The virulence factors associated with *V. vulnificus* include a capsule, cytolysin, protease/elastase and phospholipase, but these are found in nearly all clinical and environmental strains (Strom and Paranjpye, 2000). Virulence appears to be multifaceted and is not well understood, thus all strains are considered virulent.

Foodborne *V. vulnificus* infection is clearly associated with underlying medical conditions (Strom and Paranjpye, 2000). Liver disease is a prominent risk factor for *V. vulnificus* infection, including cirrhosis due to alcohol consumption. Additional risk factors include diabetes, gastrointestinal disorders (surgery, ulcers), haematological conditions, and immunodeficiency due to underlying conditions such as cancer and treatment of chronic conditions with immunosuppressive agents (e.g. arthritis). *V. vulnificus* may pose a small risk to otherwise "healthy" individuals since a small fraction of cases (<5%) are reported to occur in individuals without any identifiable risk factor. The prevalence of predisposing conditions among the adult population (>18 years of age) in the USA has been estimated in a 1997 memorandum to the FDA Office of Seafood Director (Klontz, 1997). These numbers suggest that approximately 7% of the adult population in the USA is susceptible to infection. Given the uncertainty in prevalence of liver disease (including hepatitis), this could be as high as ~16%.

*V. vulnificus* causes a mild to severe gastrointestinal illness, potentially progressing to septicaemia with a significant mortality in a susceptible population. In the USA, mortality rates are between 50% and 60% for patients with *V. vulnificus* septicaemia (Hlady and Klontz, 1996; Shapiro et al., 1998). Septicaemia is the symptom with which patients typically present to health care systems. Thus in this risk assessment septicaemia was the endpoint modelled.

This risk assessment considers only reported cases of *V. vulnificus* septicaemia from 1995 to 2001 (mean of 32 cases annually) in which a history of consumption of raw Gulf Coast oysters is documented (M. Glatzer, personal communication, 2001). Because of the severity of the septicaemia, under-reporting is not as substantial a consideration (2:1) as with gastrointestinal illnesses, which the Centers for Disease Control (CDC) estimates to have a 20:1 under-reporting ratio (Mead et al., 1999). However, various sources of under-reporting of *V. vulnificus* septicaemia have been identified. Historically, FDA has only recorded cases where patients admitted eating oysters. Patients who ate oysters may have denied oyster consumption, may not have been willing to answer questions, or may have deceased before a food history could be obtained. Another source of under-reporting is the failure to capture all the cases in different reporting systems. Adjusting for such under-reporting indicate that there may be up to 2.5 times more *V. vulnificus* septicaemia cases associated with raw Gulf Coast oysters. While this risk assessment does not make any adjustment for possible under-reporting it would be possible to do this by shifting the dose-response relationship towards greater risk at a given dose (i.e. moving the dose-response curve to the left).

There are no human volunteer studies with *V. vulnificus* from which a dose-response relationship might be estimated. Data are available to estimate the relationship by comparing monthly exposure estimates for sensitive populations with monthly-observed epidemiological data in the USA using an approach similar to that proposed by Buchanan et al. (1997). A consistent *V. vulnificus* reporting system, administered by CDC, has been in effect since 1995 in the USA, and the CDC data is currently available through to 2001.

The month- and year-specific mean *V. vulnificus* numbers at consumption were estimated based on water temperatures from 1995 through to 2001. Monthly oyster landings were found to vary less substantially from year to year than temperature. Therefore, the number of servings each month was estimated assuming that 50% of the average landings (from 1990–1998) each month are consumed raw, and then converting to a corresponding number of meals based on average oyster weight and typical number of oysters per serving. The number of meals consumed by the susceptible population was estimated as being 7% of the total meals. For the purpose of dose-response modelling, the mean *V. vulnificus* dose per serving was used to summarize group level exposures rather than the median (or other statistic) because use of the mean has been shown to minimize bias of estimated dose-response relationships from group-level data under most circumstances (Crump, 1998). Also, it is the illness burden that is the public health impact of foremost concern, which, is in turn determined by the mean (and not necessarily the median) risk per serving in respect to any given collection of (variable) exposures for which illness burden is of interest (see Appendix C). Figure 2 shows the maximum likelihood fit of the Beta-Poisson dose-response curve and the corresponding 90% confidence limits for risk of reported *V. vulnificus* illness. The dots represent the best estimates of the month- and year-specific risk per serving versus month- and year-specific estimates of average dose per serving based upon an analysis of exposure and observed epidemiology. The best estimates of parameters for the Beta-Poisson model are $\alpha = 9.3\times10^{-6}$ and $\beta = 110\ 000$.

## RISK CHARACTERIZATION

With respect to the baseline assessment, using typical seasonal water temperature parameters, the predicted mean numbers of illnesses were 0.5, 11.7, 12.2 and 8.0 for the winter (January–March), spring (April–June), summer (July–September) and autumn (October–December) seasons, respectively. These predictions were based on the seasonal estimates of mean risk per serving and the estimated number of servings consumed, and are, therefore, necessarily consistent with the observed epidemiology. Based on the dose-response assessment, the effect of alternative process target levels on risk per serving and annual cases burden was evaluated

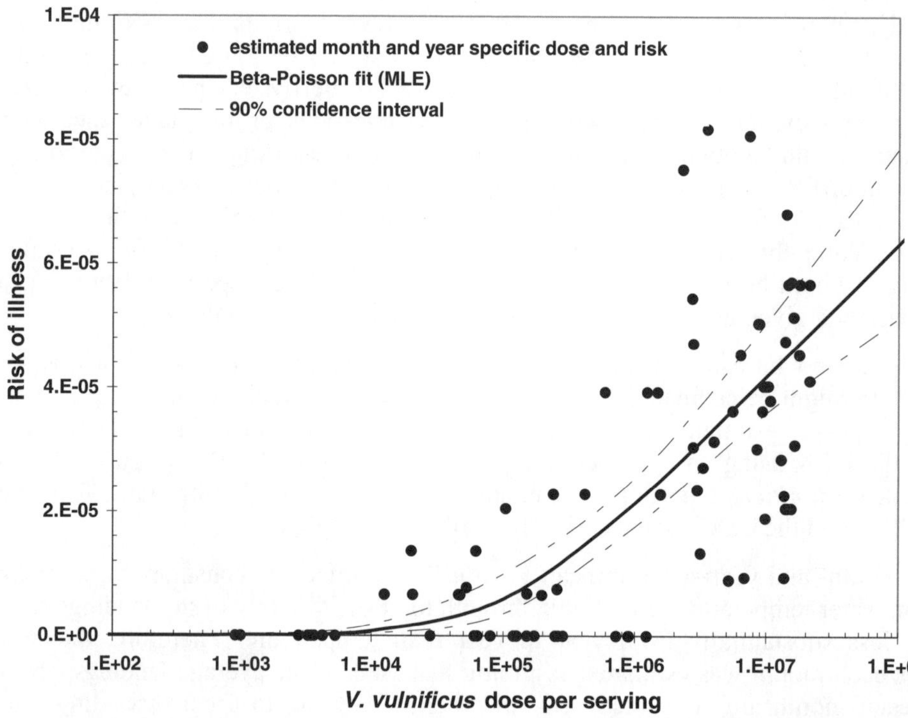


**Figure 2.** Beta-Poisson dose-response curve for *V. vulnificus* (Vv) (monthly average risk per serving versus monthly average dose per serving). Each data point is determined by risk of reported oyster-related illness (number of observed cases divided by estimated number of servings) and mean exposure corresponding to month- and year-specific water temperature data.

(Table 2). These target levels could be achieved by one or a range of intervention strategies. Substantial reductions in risk were found to be associated with target levels for *V. vulnificus* of 3/g and 30/g with an approximate 10-fold range of uncertainty. More details on the outcome and uses of this risk assessment are presented in the technical report.

**Table 2.** Predicted mean and 90% uncertainty intervals for risk per serving and annual number of illnesses for three alternative process target levels.

| Target *V. vulnificus*/g | Mean risk per serving (median and 90% interval of uncertainty distribution) | Annual number of cases (median and 90% interval of uncertainty distribution) |
|---|---|---|
| 3/g | $1.09 \times 10^{-7}$ ($4.10 \times 10^{-8}$, $2.73 \times 10^{-7}$) | 0.16 (0.06, 0.4) |
| 30/g | $8.20 \times 10^{-7}$ ($3.42 \times 10^{-7}$, $2.12 \times 10^{-6}$) | 1.2 (0.5, 3.1) |
| 300/g | $5.26 \times 10^{-6}$ ($2.60 \times 10^{-6}$, $1.05 \times 10^{-6}$) | 7.7 (3.8, 15.3) |

# CONCLUSIONS

## Key findings

- The utilization of the framework and parameters for the *V. parahaemolyticus* risk assessment facilitated the development of the *V. vulnificus* risk assessment.
- Where additional data were available it was possible to validate certain aspects of the risk assessment model. The exposure assessment predictions were validated by their close agreement with retail study data.
- In the absence of specific dose-response data it was possible to develop a dose-response relationship from exposure predictions and the reported frequency of illness which was effective for risk characterization and the evaluation of interventions.

## Limitations and caveats

In terms of applying this risk assessment to other geographical areas there are a numbers of issues which need to be specifically considered and perhaps adjusted to take into account the local situation.

- The *V. vulnificus*-temperature relationship in oysters at harvest may not be applicable to other regions or countries with different environmental conditions, such as high salinity.
- Countries harvesting different species of oysters, and that have different post-harvest handling practices or consumption patterns, may have to adjust the model inputs to account for these differences.
- The proportion of susceptible individuals may be very different in some countries, such as those in Asia and Africa that have high prevalence of hepatitis C and HIV/AIDS, respectively, or in countries with high rates of alcoholism.

Some general limitations to this risk assessment were also identified. These were primarily linked to data limitations and the availability of additional data in the future may mean that certain aspects of the risk assessment would need to be revised.

- The dose-response relationship is based on predicted mean exposure and this was found to be sensitive to the choice of available data for the *V. vulnificus*-temperature relationship in oysters at harvest. Alternative data sets gave significantly different predictions of the variance of $\log_{10}$ densities even though the mean of $\log_{10}$ densities were similar. Since dose-response and risk characterization, by the methods adopted here, depend largely on mean values, representative estimates of population variance of $\log_{10}$ densities are necessary in order to estimate mean exposure.
- The dose-response assessment and risk characterization was based on the assumption that all strains are equally virulent and there are no seasonal or regional changes in virulence.

## Conclusion and recommendations

The approach of extending the models developed in the FDA-VPRA and FAO/WHO-VPRA to model another pathogen, *V. vulnificus*, greatly facilitated the risk assessment process. The same framework and many of the model inputs were applicable for modelling *V. vulnificus* risk in USA oysters and sufficient data was available to conduct a useful risk assessment. It was also possible to develop the model in such a way as to evaluate the potential effectiveness of various mitigation strategies in terms of reducing *V. vulnificus* levels in oysters, and ultimately the risk of illness.

This model provides a strong basis for countries wanting to undertake a risk assessment on *V. vulnificus* in oysters. However, in order to apply the model it would be important to have data relevant to that country, particularly on *V. vulnificus* numbers in seafood's associated with primary septicaemia, at harvest and the point of consumption, and to characterize the susceptible population within that country. For seafood's other than raw oysters the model would need to be altered and evaluated, although the dose-response data may be applicable to other countries.

# REFERENCES

Buchanan, R.L., Damert, W.G., Whiting, R.C. & van Schothorst, M. 1997. The use of epidemiological and food survey data to estimate a purposefully conservative dose-response relationship for *Listeria monocytogenes* levels and incidence of listeriosis. *Journal of Food Protection*, **60**: 918–922.

Buchanan, R.L., Whiting, R.C. & Damert, W.C. 1997. When is simple good enough: A comparison of the Gompertz, Baranyi, and three-phase linear models for fitting bacterial growth curves. *Food Microbiology,* **14**: 313–326.

Cook, D.W. 1997a. Refrigeration of oyster shellstock: conditions which minimize the outgrowth of *Vibrio vulnificus*. *Journal of Food Protection*, **60**: 349–352.

Cook, D.W. 1997b. Survey of oysters at first dealer level to assess the effect of the Interstate Shellfish Sanitation Conference's Interim Control Plan to reduce *Vibrio vulnificus* in oysters intended for raw consumption. U.S. Food and Drug Administration.

Cook, D.W., O'Leary, P., Hunsucker, J.C., Sloan, E.M., Bowers, J.C., Blodgett, R.J. & DePaola, A. 2002. *Vibrio vulnificus* and *Vibrio parahaemolyticus* in U.S. retail shell oysters: A national survey June 1998 to July 1999. *Journal of Food Protection*, **65**: 79–87.

Crump, K.S. 1998. On summarizing group exposures in risk assessment: Is an arithmetic mean or geometric mean more appropriate? *Risk Analysis,* **18**: 293–297.

DePaola, A., Nordstrom, J.L., Dalsgaard, A., Forslund, A., Oliver, J.D., Bates, T., Bourdade, K.L. & Gulig, P.A. 2003. Analysis of *Vibrio vulnificus* from market oysters and septicaemia cases for virulence markers. *Applied and Environmental Microbiology,* **69**: 4006–4011.

Desenclos, J.A., Klontz, K.C., Wolfe, L.E. & Hoecheri, S. 1991. The risk of *Vibrio* illness in the Florida raw oyster eating population, 1981–1988. *American Journal of Epidemiology,* **134**: 290–297.

FAO/WHO [Food and Agriculture Organization of the United Nations/World Health Organization] (in press). Risk assessment of *Vibrio parahaemolyticus* in seafood.

FDA [US Food and Drug Administration]. 2001. Draft Risk Assessment on the Public Health Impacts of *Vibrio parahaemolyticus* in Raw Molluscan Shellfish. Washington, DC: U.S. Food and Drug Administration.

Hlady, W.G. 1997. *Vibrio* infections associated with raw oyster consumption in Florida, 1981–1994. *Journal of Food Protection,* **60**: 353–357.

Hlady, W.G. & Klontz, K.C. 1996. The epidemiology of *Vibrio* infections in Florida, 1981–1993. *Journal of Infectious Diseases,* **173**: 1176–1183.

Jackson, J.K., Murphree, R.L. & Tamplin, M.L. 1997. Evidence that mortality from *Vibrio vulnificus* infection results from single strains among heterogeneous populations in shellfish. *Journal of Clinical Microbiology,* **35**: 2098–2101.

Klontz, K.C. 1997. Estimated number of persons at increased risk for *Vibrio vulnificus* septicaemia: Memorandum to Phillip C. Spiller, Director of FDA Office of Seafood. Added to this publication as Appendix E.

McCoubrey, D.J. 1996. Risk of *Vibrio vulnificus* infection following consumption of raw commercially harvested North Island oysters. MPH Thesis. The University of Auckland, New Zealand. 86 p.

Mead, P.S., Slutsker, L., Dietz, V., McGaig, L.F., Bresee, J.S., Shapiro, C., Griffin, P.M. & Tauxe, R.V. 1999. Food-related illness and death in the United States. *Emerging Infectious Diseases,* **5**: 607–625.

Motes, M.L., DePaola, A., Cook, D.W., Veazey, J.E., Hunsucker, J.C., Garthright, W.E., Blodgett, R.J. & Chirtel, S.J. 1998. Influence of water temperature and salinity on *Vibrio vulnificus* in northern Gulf and Atlantic Coast oysters (*Crassostrea virginica*). *Applied and Environmental Microbiology,* **64**: 1459–1465.

NERRS [National Estuarine Research Reserve System]. 2001. Weeks Bay, AL, temperature data (available at www.ocrm.nos.noaa.gov/nerr/welcome.html).

Nilsson, W.B., Paranjpye, R.N., DePaola, A. & Strom, M.S. 2003. Sequence polymorphism of the 16S rRNA gene of *Vibrio vulnificus* is a possible indicator of strain virulence. *Journal of Clinical Microbiology,* **41**: 442–446.

NMFS [National Marine Fisheries Service]. 1998. Fisheries Data for the United States 1990–1998. (available at www.nmfs.noaa.gov).

NOAA [National Oceanic and Atmospheric Administration]. 1999. National Climatic Data Center Global Buoy Data (available at www.ncdc.noaa.gov/oa/ncdc.html).

Scientific Committee on Veterinary Measures Relating to Public Health. 2001. Opinion of the Scientific Committee on Veterinary Measures Relating to Public Health on *Vibrio vulnificus* and *Vibrio parahaemolyticus* (in raw and undercooked seafood) (adopted on 19–20 September 2001). European Commission, Health & Consumer Protection Directorate-General, Directorate C - Scientific Opinions. 64 pp.

Shapiro, R.L., Altekruse, S., Hutwagner, S., Bishop, R., Hammond, R., Wilson, S., Ray, B., Thompson, S., Tauxe, R.V., Griffin, P.M. & *Vibrio* working group. 1998. The role of Gulf Coast oysters harvested in warmer months in *Vibrio vulnificus* infections in the United States, 1988–1996. *Journal of Infectious Diseases,* **178**: 752–759.

Strom, M.S. & Paranjpye, R.N. 2000. Epidemiology and pathogenesis of *Vibrio vulnificus. Microbes and Infection,* **2**: 177–188.

Tamplin, M.L. 1994. The seasonal occurrence of *Vibrio vulnificus* in shellfish, seawater, and sediment in United States coastal waters. Final report to Salstonstall-Kennedy Grant Program, US Department of Commerce.

# TECHNICAL REPORT

# 1. Introduction

*Vibrio vulnificus* naturally inhabits warm estuarine environments and can infect humans via wound exposure or seafood consumption. These infections are rare and generally limited to individuals with pre-existing chronic illnesses or the immunocompromised. However, *V. vulnificus* can invade through the intestinal barrier into the bloodstream (primary septicaemia) and has the highest case/fatality rate (approx. 50%) among foodborne pathogens. While *V. vulnificus* has been found in a variety of seafood's worldwide and illnesses have been reported in a number of countries, its epidemiology, ecology and distribution in seafood's have been most extensively investigated in the United States of America (USA). Each year, 30 to 40 primary septicaemia cases are reported in the USA, and nearly all are associated with consumption of raw oysters harvested from the Gulf Coast.

A risk assessment for the pathogen-commodity pair of *V. vulnificus* in raw oysters was proposed by the European Community in the 33rd session of the Codex Committee on Food Hygiene (CCFH) (CAC, 2000). There have been at least two previous risk assessments on *V. vulnificus*. McCoubrey (1996) reported on the risk of *V. vulnificus* infection following consumption of raw commercially harvested North Island oysters from New Zealand in 1996. The report concluded that environmental conditions, especially high salinities, were not suitable for *V. vulnificus* survival. The European Commission's Scientific Committee on Veterinary Measures relating to Public Health has prepared a document on *V. vulnificus* and *V. parahaemolyticus* in raw and undercooked seafood (Scientific Committee on Veterinary Measures relating to Public Health, 2001). This work followed the general format of a risk assessment and noted variations in *V. vulnificus* prevalence on a global scale. However, neither of the above risk assessments was quantitative. In order to address the risk associated with *V. vulnificus* in a quantitative manner, within the framework of the FAO/WHO risk assessment on *Vibrio* spp. in seafood, it was decided to extend the *V. parahaemolyticus* models described in the U.S. Food and Drug Administration (USFDA) Draft Risk Assessment on the Public Health Impacts of *V. parahaemolyticus* in Raw Molluscan Shellfish ("FDA-VPRA") (FDA, 2001) and the Joint FAO/WHO Risk Assessment of *V. parahaemolyticus* in Raw Oysters ("FAO/WHO-VPRA") (FAO/WHO, in press) to *V. vulnificus.* The general approach proposed and many of the parameters used in the present *V. vulnificus* risk assessment are the same as those used in the FDA-VPRA and FAO/WHO-VPRA.

## 1.1. Scope

This risk assessment had several objectives. Firstly, it aimed to determine the usefulness of adapting the FDA-VPRA and FAO/WHO-VPRA models to assess the risk from *V. vulnificus* septicaemia associated with the consumption of raw oysters. Secondly, the risk assessment aimed to identify the most appropriate data, as well as gaps in the available dataset, for modelling purposes. In addition to estimating the risk of *V. vulnificus* septicaemia associated with the consumption of raw oysters, the risk assessment model was also developed with the objective of evaluating targeted mitigation levels aimed at reducing the risk of *V. vulnificus* septicaemia. For reasons of data availability, the risk assessment was limited to consideration of primary septicaemia cases associated with consumption of raw oysters from the Gulf Coast of the United States of America (USA).

A number of factors facilitated the development of this risk assessment of *V. vulnificus* in raw oysters and served to reduce the amount of work needed to complete the risk assessment. These included the following:

1. A history of consistent active surveillance in the USA and a much higher reporting rate for primary septicaemia (>50%) compared with low and highly variable reporting for gastrointestinal infections.
2. A well characterized seasonal effect that relates exposure to frequency of *V. vulnificus* illness.
3. The dominance of a single vehicle of transmission (>90% of cases of illness are associated with the consumption raw Gulf Coast oysters).
4. The storage of oysters in the shell until consumption practically eliminates potential for cross-contamination, thereby reducing uncertainty.
5. Raw consumption eliminates variability and uncertainty on pathogen survival during preparation, in contrast to the diverse cooking procedures used with other commodities.
6. The availability of extensive quantitative data on levels of *V. vulnificus* in oysters at harvest and at the point of consumption.
7. Information on the growth and survival of natural *V. vulnificus* populations in oysters under typical industry practices from harvest to consumption.
8. The availability of the USFDA Draft Risk Assessment on the Public Health Impacts of *V. parahaemolyticus* in Raw Molluscan Shellfish (FDA, 2001) and the Joint FAO/WHO Risk Assessment of *V. parahaemolyticus* in Raw Oysters (in preparation), which provide a suitable framework and many of the necessary parameters formatted for risk assessment, thereby also reducing the work to be undertaken.
9. The tagging system for USA oysters which permits tracing of harvest dates and locations.

The current risk assessment establishes a relationship for predicting *V. vulnificus* levels at harvest based on seasonal and yearly variations of water temperature. Distributions of storage times and temperatures representative of industry practices are used to predict growth and survival post-harvest. These distributions along with surveyed oyster consumption patterns are used to determine exposure to *V. vulnificus*. Predicted exposure is validated using data from a national market survey of *V. vulnificus* in raw oysters. Hazard characterization relies primarily on a dose-response relationship derived from the seasonal relationship of predicted exposure and reported illness frequencies. This dose-response relationship is used to predict illness frequencies at targeted mitigation levels that may be achieved through various interventions.

# 2. Hazard identification

Since *V. vulnificus* was first reported in the 1970s, it has been the subject of many research and review articles (Oliver, 1989; Strom and Paranjpye, 2000). Three biotypes of *V. vulnificus* have been reported (Bisharat and Raz, 1997; Bisharat et al., 1999): Biotype 1 accounts for nearly all human cases resulting from seafood consumption, whereas Biotype 2 is associated with infections in cultured eels and Biotype 3 has been limited to wound infections associated with handling fish cultured in inland ponds in Israel. Most of the studies of Biotype 1 *V. vulnificus* have been conducted in the USA, and outside of that country there is currently little epidemiological information as *V. vulnificus* is not a reportable disease in most countries and surveillance is limited. While foodborne *V. vulnificus* infections are relatively rare in the USA (approximately 30–40 reported cases of primary septicaemia per year), they have the highest case fatality ratio among foodborne illnesses, which exceeds 50% (Hlady and Klontz, 1996; Mead et al., 1999; M. Glatzer, personal communication, 2001). Individuals with pre-existing liver disease are at greatest risk of contracting primary septicaemia, with subsequent mortality, but other chronic illnesses and immune deficiency conditions are also associated with increased risk. Healthy individuals may be at risk for relatively mild gastroenteritis, which is outside the scope of this assessment, but the risk for primary septicaemia in the absence of reported risk factors is considered negligible.

A number of factors have been reported as possible virulence determinants in *V. vulnificus*, including an extracellular cytolysin, protease, siderophores, a phospholipase, polysaccharide capsule, resistance to bactericidal effects of human serum, resistance to phagocytosis, and the ability to acquire iron from transferrin (Oliver, 1989; Strom and Paranjpye, 2000). The relevance of these factors has been examined in various *in vivo* or *in vitro* models. Production of disease by this bacterium appears to be multifaceted, involving a variety of virulence attributes and host susceptibility factors. Most animal studies have not found major differences in virulence characteristics between clinical and environmental isolates of *V. vulnificus* (Table 1). However, this is inconsistent with the low attack rate in susceptible populations consuming seafood contaminated with *V. vulnificus*. Less than one illness occurs per 10 000 meals of raw Gulf oysters served to the highest risk population, people with liver diseases (Hlady, 1994), suggesting that environmental strains are not equally virulent or not all people with liver disease are equally susceptible.

Nearly all *V. vulnificus* primary septicaemia cases in the USA have been associated with consumption of raw oysters harvested from the Gulf Coast. These cases follow a seasonal distribution, with approximately 90% of cases occurring from April through November (M. Glatzer, personal communication, 2001). Only one confirmed foodborne case has been associated with oysters harvested other than from the Gulf Coast, and only two cases have been linked to oysters harvested in January or February. The seasonal numbers of *V. vulnificus* in Gulf Coast oysters at harvest (Motes et al., 1998; Tamplin, 1994) and at retail (Cook et al., 2002) exhibit a similar distribution to the cases of *V. vulnificus* illness.

**Table 1.** Summary of virulence testing from clinical and environmental *V. vulnificus* strains using various animal models.

| Model | Dose/Route(3) | No. virulent/No. of isolates tested | | Reference |
|---|---|---|---|---|
| | | Clinical strains | Environmental strains | |
| Normal adult mouse | $10^6$/i.p. | 2/3 | Not tested | Poole and Oliver, 1978 |
| Normal adult mouse | $10^6$/s.c. | 2/3 | Not tested | Poole and Oliver, 1978 |
| Normal adult mouse | $10^8$/i.v. | 1/1 | Not tested | Poole and Oliver, 1978 |
| Normal adult mouse | $10^8$/o.g. | 0/1 | Not tested | Poole and Oliver, 1978 |
| Normal adult mouse | $10^8$/i.p. | 20/20 | 25/29 | Tison and Kelly, 1986 |
| Normal adult mouse | $10^8$/i.p. | 4/4 | 40/40 | Kaysner et al., 1987 |
| Normal adult mouse | $10^6$/i.p. | 7/11 | 9/13 | Stelma et al., 1992 |
| Iron-overload mouse(1) | $10^0$/i.p. | 1/1 | Not tested | Wright, Simpson and Oliver, 1981 |
| Iron-overload mouse(1) | $10^3$/i.p. | 4/8 | 2/8 | Morris et al., 1987 |
| Iron-overload mouse(2) | $10^2$/i.p. | 3/4 | 4/7 | Kaysner et al., 1987 |
| Iron-overload mouse(2) | $10^2$/i.p. | 8/11 | 9/13 | Stelma et al., 1992 |
| Iron-overload mouse(2) | $10^3$/i.p. | 1/1 | 1/8 | Jackson, Murphree and Tamplin, 1997 |
| Iron-overload and immuno-compromised mouse | $10^3$/i.p. | 0/3 | 4/4 | Stelma et al., 1992 |
| Suckling mouse | $10^6$/o.g. | 5/5 | 0/7 | Johnson et al., 1984 |
| Suckling mouse | $10^7$/o.g. | 4/8 | 2/8 | Morris et al., 1987 |
| Suckling mouse | $10^5$/o.g. | 5/6 | 2/5 | Reyes et al., 1987 |

NOTES: (1) Ferric ammonium citrate (80 mg/kg) used to produce iron-overload. (2) Iron dextran (250 mg/kg) used to produce iron-overload. (3) Route of administration (i.p. = intraperitoneal injection; s.c. = subcutaneous injection; i.v. = intravenous injection; o.g. = orogastric ingestion).

# 3. Exposure assessment

## 3.1. Microbial ecology

*Vibrio vulnificus* is a bacterium that occurs naturally in estuaries in many parts of the world (Oliver, 1989). Its distribution and abundance is affected by temperature and salinity of the seawater. *V. vulnificus* is present in waters, sediments, plankton, molluscs, crustaceans and finfish estuaries of the Gulf Coast of the USA (Tamplin, 1990; DePaola, Capers and Alexander, 1994). A recent study in India highlighted the presence of *V. vulnificus* in the tropical waters of the southwest coast of India (Parvathi et al., 2004).

Attention is generally focused on oysters, since most *V. vulnificus*-related foodborne illnesses in the USA are linked to their raw consumption. *V. vulnificus* is found in various tissues of the oyster and may reside within oyster haemocytes (Tamplin and Capers, 1992; Harris-Young et al., 1993). Each oyster may shed up to one million *V. vulnificus* cells per day into the water, demonstrating its ability to multiply within the oyster (Tamplin and Capers, 1992).

Typically, USA Gulf Coast oysters harbour about 1000 *V. vulnificus* cells per gram during the warmer months of April through to October, and usually less than 10 per gram during other months, although *V. vulnificus* may become undetectable in Gulf Coast oysters during unusually cold periods (DePaola, Capers and Alexander, 1994; Motes et al., 1998). Oysters from the southwest coast of India were found to harbour *V. vulnificus* at a level of 1000 per gram when water salinity was at its lowest, during and after the monsoon (Parvathi et al., 2004). At other times of the year, when water salinity was more than 25 ppt, less than 10 cells per gram were detected. Some evidence suggests that this bacterium lives in oysters year round but may become dormant or viable but non-culturable (VBNC) during cold weather; a temporary condition reversible by increasing water temperature (Nilsson, Oliver and Kjelleberg, 1991). *V. vulnificus* numbers in seawater are approximately 100-fold lower than in oysters, but numbers frequently exceed $10^6$ per gram in the intestines of bottom feeding fish that inhabit oyster reefs (DePaola, Capers and Alexander, 1994).

Unlike many shellfish-borne human pathogens, *V. vulnificus* is not associated with human faeces and traditional indicators of faecal pollution (i.e. faecal coliforms) are not effective at predicting its abundance in oysters (Tamplin et al., 1982). A number of factors may interact with temperature and salinity to control *V. vulnificus* populations in oysters, including nutrient availability, resuspension of sediments, plankton blooms, defecation by vertebrates (i.e. finfish), phagocytosis by oyster haemocytes, competition, predation, phage infections and a variety of physical factors (pH, dissolved oxygen, water chemistry and sunlight). The effect of these factors on *V. vulnificus* ecology is unknown, making the prospect of developing a reliable indicator model in the near future extremely unlikely.

## 3.2. Growth and survival characteristics

The bacterium may grow at temperatures as low as 13°C (Kaspar and Tamplin, 1993), but its numbers in the environment remain low at temperatures below 20°C (Kelly, 1982; O'Neill, Jones and Grimes, 1992). Highest concentrations occur when the water temperature is between 20°C and 30°C. Thus, *V. vulnificus* is more abundant along the Gulf Coast than in the cooler waters of the Atlantic and Pacific Coasts of the USA (DePaola, Capers and Alexander, 1994; Cook, 1994; Tamplin, 1990; O'Neill, Jones and Grimes, 1992; Kaysner et al., 1987; Motes et al., 1998). *V. vulnificus* can be found at salinities ranging from 0.8 to 35 ppt (Tamplin, 1990; Kaysner et al., 1987). The salinity optimum for *V. vulnificus* appears to vary considerably from area to area, but highest numbers are usually found at intermediate salinities of 5 to 25 ppt (Tamplin et al., 1982; Kelly, 1982; O'Neill, Jones and Grimes, 1992; Tamplin, 1990; Motes et al., 1998).

*V. vulnificus* is more sensitive than other *Vibrio* spp. and most other foodborne pathogens to most inactivation techniques used in food processing. A mild heat treatment of 50°C for 5 minutes yielded a 6 $\log_{10}$ reduction in *V. vulnificus* in shucked oyster meats (Cook and Ruple, 1992). Freezing oysters at -40°C and storage for 3 weeks achieved a 4 to 5 $\log_{10}$ reduction in the natural *V. vulnificus* population (Cook and Ruple, 1992). However, the effectiveness of freezing may be reduced in *V. vulnificus* cells subjected to a cold adaptation step of 15°C prior to freezing (Bryan et al., 1999). Similar reductions can be readily achieved by irradiation (Ama, Hamdy and Toledo, 1994) and high hydrostatic pressure (Berlin et al., 1999). Low pH is quite lethal to *V. vulnificus* (Koo, Marshall and DePaola, 2001), but organisms within the oyster tissues may be protected from acidic hot sauces and other chemicals as these would probably not penetrate to the interior of an oyster (Sun and Oliver, 1994, 1995). Depuration was shown not to be effective in elimination of *V. vulnificus* as it resides within various oyster tissues, but relaying oysters to high salinity waters (>32 ppt) was shown to reduce *V. vulnificus* numbers by 3–4 logs (<10 per g) within 2 weeks (Motes and DePaola, 1996).

## 3.3. Consumption of oysters

Intake data for molluscan shellfish are available from a number of governmental and non-governmental sources, but the information in the data is sometimes limited. In many countries there is a scarcity of such consumption data, as noted recently in the European Union (Scientific Committee on Veterinary Measures relating to Public Health, 2001). Because raw shellfish is not a commonly consumed food in many countries, including the USA (10–20% of the population consumes shellfish raw at least once during a year), the available data from nationwide general nutrition surveys generally do not provide definitive information as to consumption patterns. For example, data from the U.S. Department of Agriculture (USDA) Continuing Survey of Food Intake by Individuals (CFSII) (USDA/ARS, various dates) suggest that, over the aggregate USA population, raw oysters are consumed on average at a rate of 0.0005 servings per person per day, with a mean serving size of 110 grams. While this rate of consumption is based on a relatively large number of survey respondents (~15 000), the estimate of serving size from the same data is much more uncertain. It is based on the consumption behaviour of only 6 individuals reporting consumption during the survey period.

Another food frequency survey, which was specific to raw oyster consumption in the state of Florida in the USA, was conducted by the Agricultural Market Research Center, University of Florida (Degner and Petrone, 1994). This study was judged to provide substantially better information with respect to the probable distribution of serving sizes and, though regional, was considered more appropriate as an estimate of the national consumption patterns, bearing in mind the limited number of individuals reporting oyster consumption in the larger (national) surveys. The data from the Florida survey indicate a distribution of serving sizes with a mean of ~13.7 oysters/serving. Combining these data with oyster weight data obtained during a retail study (Cook et al., 2002; A. DePaola, personal communication, 2002) suggests a mean serving size of ~196 g. Based on this estimate of average serving size, the total number of servings consumed can be determined from landings data (NMFS, 1998) and an estimate of the percentage of the harvest that is consumed raw.

This is the approach to estimation of consumption behaviour (number of servings and size of serving) that was used in the FDA-VPRA and the FAO/WHO-VPRA and was taken from that work for the purpose of this assessment. Since the current risk assessment is restricted to consideration of risk associated with USA Gulf Coast oysters, only oysters harvested from that specific region were considered here.

## 3.4. Modelling exposure to *V. vulnificus*

A schematic diagram of the *V. vulnificus* risk assessment model is shown in Figure 1. Modelling exposure to *V. vulnificus* followed the same approach and used many of the same assumptions as used for the FAO/WHO-VPRA (FAO/WHO, in press) and FDA-VPRA (FDA, 2001). These are summarized in Table 2. While foodborne *V. vulnificus* infections have been reported in countries other than the USA, such as Taiwan (Chuang et al., 1992) and the Republic of Korea (Park, Shon and Joh, 1991), sufficient data are currently available only in the USA for most of the model inputs shown in Figure 1. This framework could be used by other countries to model the risk of *V. vulnificus* illness from raw oysters when the appropriate data is available. It may also be modified to address other seafood's.

The production-process-retail-consumption continuum was modelled using a modular approach. Each of the modules – harvest, post-harvest including storage, and retail – and the data sources for each are outlined in the following sections. For each identified step in the process continuum, variability distributions or quantitative relationships, or both, between variables were estimated based on the available data. Where applicable, uncertainties associated with these distributions and relationships were quantified. The estimated variability and uncertainty distributions and their interdependences were then implemented using Monte Carlo modelling software in order to calculate model-based exposure predictions and associated uncertainties (see Appendix A).

### 3.4.1. Harvest

#### 3.4.1.1. Water temperature and salinity distributions

Like *V. parahaemolyticus*, the numbers of *V. vulnificus* at harvest are influenced predominantly by water temperatures and salinities. Other factors may also contribute to *V. vulnificus* numbers, but only the effects of temperature and salinity have been quantified (Motes et al., 1998).

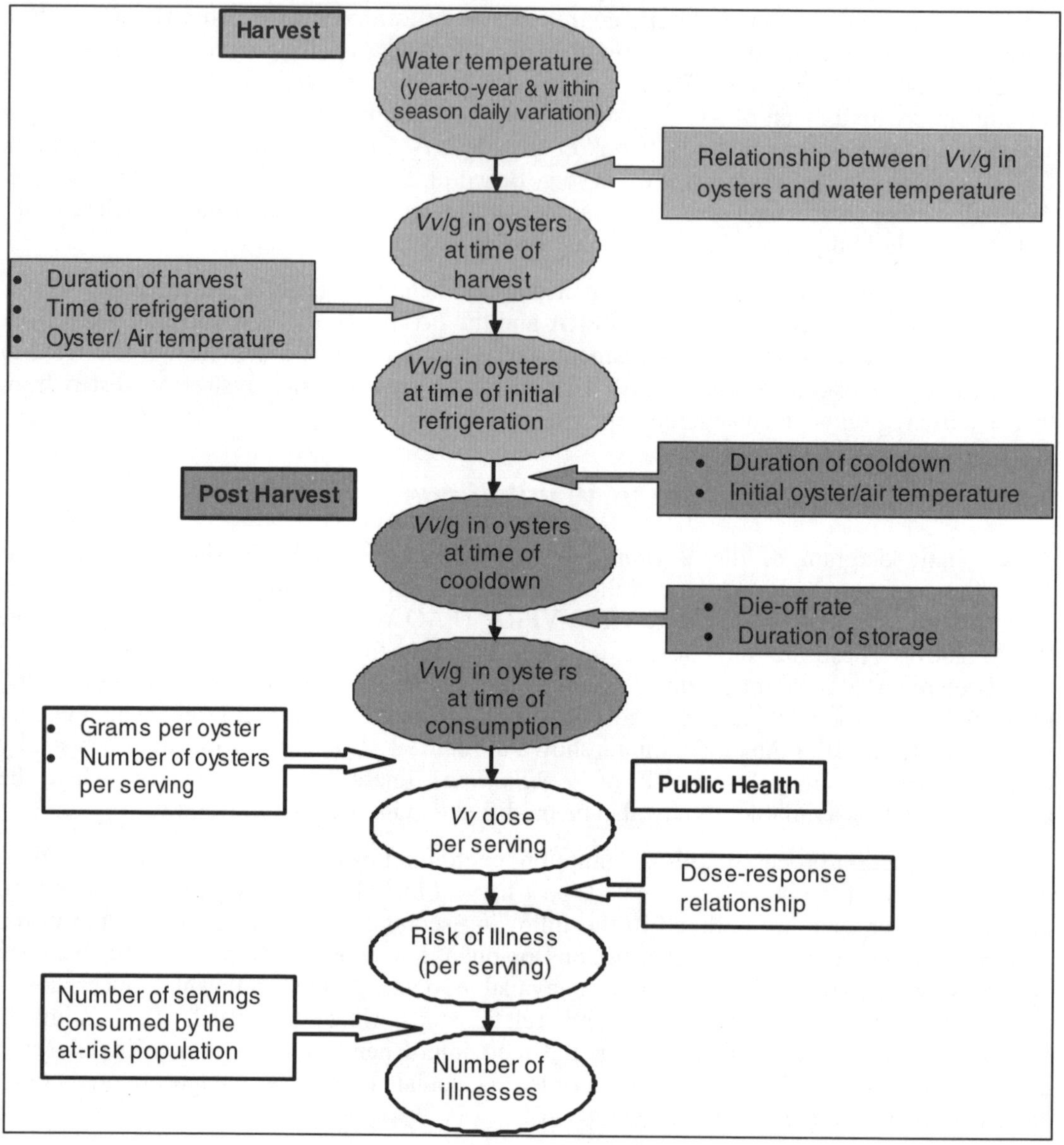


**Figure 1**. Schematic diagram of the *V. vulnificus* (Vv) conceptual risk assessment model, showing integration of all modules.

**Table 2**. Model inputs, data sources and assumptions for the proposed *V. vulnificus* risk assessment

| Model Inputs | Data Source | Assumptions |
|---|---|---|
| Water temperature | FAO/WHO-VPRA/FDA-VPRA; NOAA buoy data (NOAA, 1999); and NERRS (NERRS, 2001) | Buoy and other fixed site data are representative of growing areas. |
| Total *V. vulnificus* numbers at harvest | Weekly oyster samples from 4 Gulf States 1994–1995 (Motes et al., 1998; Tamplin, 1994) | Data relevant for other years. |
| Pathogenic *V. vulnificus* numbers at harvest | Weekly oyster samples from 4 Gulf States 1994–1995 (Motes et al., 1998; Tamplin, 1994) | All *V. vulnificus* strains are equally virulent. Data from Jackson, Murphree and Tamplin (1997) and two recent studies (Nilsson et al., 2003; DePaola et al., 2003) suggest opposing view on this subject, but neither addresses seasonal or regional differences in virulence. |
| Air temperature | FAO/WHO-VPRA/FDA-VPRA; NOAA buoy data (NOAA, 1999) | Temperature of oyster meat equilibrates rapidly to that of air. |
| Time harvest vessel in water | FAO/WHO-VPRA/FDA-VPRA; Dealer survey (Cook, 1997b) | Harvest practices have not changed since 1996. |
| Time to first refrigeration | FAO/WHO-VPRA/FDA-VPRA; Dealer survey (Cook, 1997b) | Oysters are harvested at a constant rate throughout the harvest period. |
| *V. vulnificus* growth rate | Natural populations in oysters at ambient temperature (Cook, 1997a). Data lacking at lower temperature | *V. vulnificus* grows at similar temperature-specific rates in Gulf oysters from April to October. |
| *V. vulnificus*/g at first refrigeration | Dealer survey of Gulf oysters 1995–1996 (Cook, 1997b) | Dealer practices in 1996 are typical of current practices. |
| Cool down time | FAO/WHO-VPRA/FDA-VPRA; no data | Rectangular (uniform) distribution between 1 and 10 h. |
| *V. vulnificus*/g at cool down | Dealer survey of Gulf oysters 1995–1996 (Cook, 1997b) | Dealer practices in 1996 are typical of current practices. |
| *V. vulnificus* survival | Natural populations in oysters stored at 3°C for 14-17 d (Cook et al., 2002) | *V. vulnificus* die off at 3°C similar to that at other temperatures between 0-13°C. |
| Pathogenic *V. vulnificus*/g at consumption | Retail study of USA oysters 1998–1999 (Cook et al., 2002) | Data are relevant for other years. (The autumn of 1998 was extremely warm and *V. vulnificus* levels were considerably higher than levels predicted for typical autumn temperatures). |
| Percentage of population susceptible | Prevalence of liver disease, immune disorder, etc., in the USA (Klontz, 1997; Desenclos et al., 1991; Shapiro et al., 1998; Hlady, 1997) | All predisposing conditions have been identified and risk of infection is homogeneous with respect to these conditions. There is no risk of illness (septicaemia) to individuals without the identified disease conditions. |
| Percentage of oysters consumed raw | 50% oysters consumed raw; FAO/WHO-VPRA | Susceptible individuals consume raw oysters at the same rate as the total population. |
| No. of oysters per serving | FAO/WHO-VPRA/FDA-VPRA | Consumption behaviour has not changed appreciably in recent years. |
| Weight per oyster | Retail study of USA oysters 1998–1999 (Cook et al., 2002) | None. |
| Risk of illness | Relationship between monthly exposure and illness within defined (Gulf States) population (Cook et al., 2002; M. Glatzer, personal communication, 2001; NMFS, 1998) | Consumption of raw oysters among the susceptible population does not vary from month to month. (If the percentage of raw oysters consumed was greater in cooler months, the effect of the assumption would be to over-predict the risk at lower *V. vulnificus* levels).<br>Reporting of *V. vulnificus* septicaemia cases related to oyster consumption does not vary from month to month. |
| Number of illnesses | Risk of illness (from above) multiplied by number of servings | Same as above for risk of illness. |

The FAO/WHO-VPRA did not quantify the distribution of salinities prevalent in growing areas. It was noted that there was little systematic collection of salinity data outside of a few selected estuaries (e.g. sites within the National Estuarine Research Reserve System – NERRS – within the USA), and that what data was available was relatively recent and did not quantify extremes of salinities that might be expected over longer periods. Water temperature data was obtained from the National Buoy Data Center (NOAA) for sites considered representative of selected regions in the USA. For the purposes of this exposure assessment, the FAO/WHO-VPRA and FDA-VPRA water temperature distributions for the USA Gulf Coast based on the NOAA data were used. However, this was supplemented by additional data from a nearby NERRS site (NERRS, 2001) for selected periods during which, due to instrument malfunction, data was not available from the NOAA temperature record.

Seasonal exposure assessments were performed for the Gulf Coast. The water temperature in the summer averages 28.9°C and varies from day to day, with a standard deviation of 1.5°C. The corresponding average and standard deviation in the winter are 14.2°C and 2.7°C, respectively. Spring and autumn are typically transitional periods with greater month-to-month variability. The temperature parameters (mean and standard deviation of day-to-day variations) within any given season vary from year to year, as discussed in the FAO/WHO-VPRA, and this variation was incorporated into the present exposure assessment.

The effect of salinity on predicted *V. vulnificus* numbers merits particular consideration. Effects of salinities on *V. vulnificus* may be stronger than on *V. parahaemolyticus* and lack of comprehensive season-specific and harvest-area-specific salinity data presents a potential data gap. While salinities >30 ppt are unusual in commercial oyster growing areas along the USA Gulf Coast, they are typical of many growing areas both in other parts of the USA and many other countries and are generally associated with low or non-detectable levels of *V. vulnificus* regardless of temperature.

There appears to be a threshold salinity level (i.e. at or slightly above 30 ppt) at which point *V. vulnificus* levels drop substantially, regardless of temperature. This abrupt change in *V. vulnificus* levels relative to salinity and the observation of a large proportion of non-detectable levels at high salinities makes quantitative estimation of the joint effects of salinity and temperature problematic over the entire range of both moderate and high salinity. Consequently, prediction of *V. vulnificus* levels has been addressed separately for high versus moderate (or low) salinity. It should be noted that the incremental effect of salinity within the moderate salinity range (i.e. <30 ppt) is not, ostensibly, the same as the effect at high salinity.

#### 3.4.1.2. Prediction of the distribution of at-harvest *V. vulnificus* numbers at moderate salinities (<30 ppt)

Levels of *V. vulnificus* in USA Gulf Coast oysters at harvest have been investigated in a number of studies (Tamplin et al., 1982; Motes et al., 1998; Vanoy, Tamplin and Schwartz, 1992; Jackson, Murphree and Tamplin, 1997). The study by Motes et al. (1998) examined *V. vulnificus* numbers in three major Gulf Coast estuaries at weekly intervals for 15 months and was selected for the exposure assessment as samples were collected more intensively and extensively than in previous studies (Motes et al., 1998 – hereafter referred to simply as the Motes et al. study). The enumeration procedures used in this study were the same as those used for other model inputs in this exposure assessment such as examinations of market oysters for levels of the pathogen and determining *V. vulnificus* growth and survival.

Additional data on *V. vulnificus* levels in oysters at harvest were provided to the risk assessment drafting group by Dr Mark Tamplin. These data were collected weekly or fortnightly from selected sites on the Gulf, Pacific and Atlantic Coasts from 1994 and 1995. The method of enumeration was comparable to that of the Motes et al. study. *V. vulnificus* levels in samples collected from Gulf Coast sites in the Tamplin (1994) study were found to be generally consistent with the observations of Motes et al. in regard to mean $\log_{10}$ levels but with substantially more variability around the mean $\log_{10}$ levels. The data collected outside of the Gulf Coast were from relatively cold water sites and *V. vulnificus* levels were frequently found to be below the limit of detection (0.3 MPN/g). These data were consistent with the observed *V. vulnificus* levels in Gulf Coast samples collected at similarly low temperatures but, due to the censoring at the limit of detection, these data provide limited information with respect to estimating a quantitative relationship between *V. vulnificus* levels and water temperature.

Like *V. parahaemolyticus*, ambient water temperatures and salinities influence *V. vulnificus* numbers at harvest (Oliver, Warner and Cleland, 1982; Motes et al., 1998). Correlation statistics indicate that temperature and salinity account for about 60% to 70% of the total variation of observed *V. vulnificus* numbers (Motes et al., 1998). The effect of salinity was found to be significant, with the $R^2$ of a temperature-only regression model being 0.60 in comparison with an $R^2$ of 0.70 when the effects of salinity were added to the regression model (Motes et al., 1998). This suggests that, after temperature, effects of salinity explain an additional 10% of the total variation of *V. vulnificus* numbers observed in the USA Gulf Coast. Other factors may influence the regional and seasonal variation but there is insufficient information available at present for the purpose of quantitative modelling.

Given the limited information in the Tamplin data collected outside of the Gulf Coast, only the data collected from Gulf Coast sites was evaluated further. These data (referred to hereafter as the "Tamplin study data") were considered together with the data from the Motes et al. study to evaluate and estimate the effects of temperature (and salinity) on *V. vulnificus* levels. Following the approach of Motes et al., standard (so-called "fixed effect") polynomial regression models were used. These models assume homogeneous residual variation around fitted regression lines. Consequently, given that *V. vulnificus* levels are observed to be unevenly distributed (i.e. positively skewed) densities were log-transformed to normalize the variance and obtain a response variable consistent with the modelling assumptions underlying use of these standard regression methods.

Additionally, in the Tamplin data, *V. vulnificus* was frequently non-detectable at low to moderately low temperatures (i.e. near or below 15°C). Such measurement outcomes are said to be censored at the limit of detection and "censored"-regression likelihoods are appropriate for obtaining parameter estimates from such data when the proportion of non-detects is high or otherwise unduly influential. Given the frequency of non-detects observed in the Tamplin data at low temperature, this approach was judged to be appropriate and was adopted here. In comparison, very few samples in the Motes et al. study had non-detectable levels. On only two occasions were the levels of *V. vulnificus* below the limit of detection in each of two replicate samples analysed per sampling occasion. When only one of the two replicates had non-detectable levels in the Motes et al. study, the MPN estimate of the sample with a detectable level was taken as the estimate corresponding to the sampling occasion, and the geometric mean was used when both replicates had detectable levels. On the two occasions when both replicates had non-detectable levels, the level corresponding to the sampling occasion was considered censored. The limit of detection for both the Tamplin and the Motes et al. studies was 0.3 MPN/g.

The polynomial regression model(s) used to examine and summarize temperature effects based on the two available data sets was of the general (quadratic) form:

$$\log(Vv/g) = \alpha + \beta_1 * Temp + \beta_2 * Temp^2 + \varepsilon$$
$$\varepsilon \sim Normal(0,\sigma^2)$$

In this equation the parameters $\alpha$, $\beta_1$, and $\beta_2$ determine the regression line (or curve) and $\varepsilon$ is the random residual (unexplained) variation, assumed to be independent of temperature and normally distributed with variance $\sigma^2$. When considering effects of salinity (below), a similar quadratic effect (in salinity) was added to the temperature-only model (above). Statistical significance of parameter estimates were examined to determine whether or not the quadratic model provided a significant improvement over the usual linear model (i.e. $\beta_2$ equal to zero).

In the process of evaluating the appropriateness of the fit of models to the available data, the model was fitted to the Motes et al. and Tamplin data sets separately; and then to the Motes et al. and Tamplin data combined (see Appendix B). Comparison of the results of these model fits to the data sets separately and combined indicated substantial differences, which could not be reconciled in the context of the regression model being used to summarize the information in these data (see Appendix B). This finding indicated that it was not appropriate to simply combine data, on an equal basis, into a single (pooled) data set within the context of the selected model(s). The implications of this can be somewhat problematic from a modelling or statistical perspective. As noted by one reviewer, when data sets are pooled and discrepancies are then identified in statistical analyses, this may be taken as an indication that the model being fitted to the data is mis-specified. That is, one may be able to identify other types of equally plausible models that effectively explain and account for the appearance of divergent characteristics in data obtained from different studies. Such statistical models and methods, when applied to data combined from multiple studies, are generally referred to as being “meta-analyses”.

As is the case with all types of statistical analysis, meta-analysis of pooled data to model (or estimate) common effects (i.e. temperature) and study-specific effects should be grounded on a plausible rationale. That is, models selected to summarize the data or to account for apparent differences between studies or both, should be sensible and understandable. However, given limited information, this can not always be satisfactorily achieved. This, it was judged, is the case here. A plausible and sensible “meta-analytic” model that would explain the apparent and substantial differences between the Tamplin versus Motes et al. data sets was not identified. In the absence of such a model, the divergence of results obtained from these multiple analyses with different data sets (i.e. separately versus pooled) was considered an uncertainty and this uncertainty was propagated through the risk assessment (see Appendix D) to fully evaluate its effect. The outcome of comparing these results indicated that exposure predictions based on the Motes et al. data were more consistent with data available for validation, and this is discussed further below, as well as in Appendix D. Thus, it was concluded that the “best estimate” of the relationship between water temperature and *V. vulnificus* levels in oysters at harvest was associated with estimates obtained by analysis of the Motes et al. data alone.

The maximum likelihood estimate (MLE) of a temperature-only regression of the quadratic form based on the Motes et al. Gulf Coast data alone is shown in Figure 2. The data shown in the figure are the averaged MPN determinations of the two replicate samples collected per each sampling occasion during this study.

In fitting the model to these data, the quadratic effect ($\beta_2$) was found to be a significant improvement over that of a linear regression model, as there is evident plateauing of *V. vulnificus* levels at temperatures above 25°C. Predictions of mean $\log_{10}$ *V. vulnificus* numbers based on this fitted regression were judged appropriate in the range of temperature from 10°C up to ~32°C (i.e. up to but not beyond the maximum of the quadratic). Similar analysis of the Tamplin data alone indicated that the quadratic (i.e. plateauing) effect at higher temperatures was not significant (see Appendix B). The MLEs of the parameters of the fit to the Motes et al. data are:

$$\alpha = -5.66$$
$$\beta_1 = 0.56$$
$$\beta_2 = -0.0086$$
$$\sigma = 0.73$$

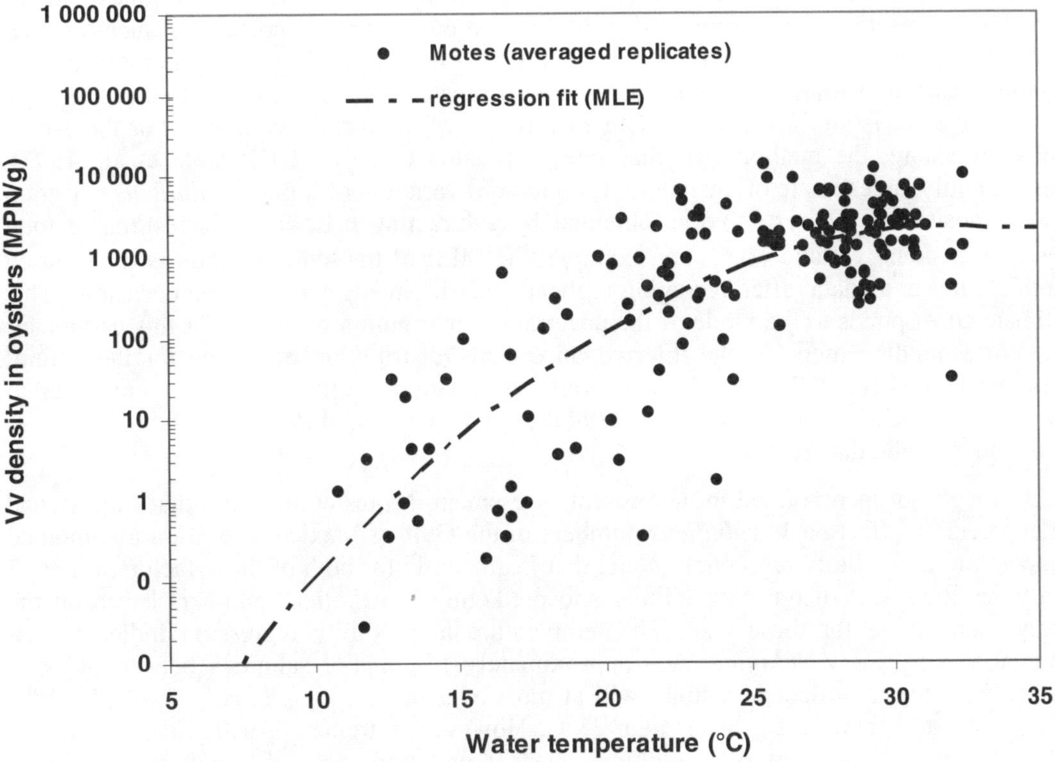


**Figure 2.** *Vibrio vulnificus* (Vv) numbers in USA Gulf Coast Oysters. Data from Motes et al., 1998.

The estimates of regression parameters based on fitting the same model to the Tamplin data set alone and then to pooled data from both studies are given in Appendix B. Additionally, with respect to all of these analyses, the uncertainty associated with the MLEs of the parameters of the regression model fits was characterized by the asymptotic variance-covariance of the parameter estimates. This is a large sample "normal approximation" of the uncertainty of the parameter values consistent with the observed data. This approximation was judged appropriate given 160 sampling occasions (and duplicate samples per sampling occasion) in the Motes et al. study and a comparable number of sampling occasions in the Tamplin study. Thus, when incorporating model estimates of the temperature effect into model simulations of exposure, the variance-covariance matrices of the parameter estimates were used (together with the MLEs) to generate uncertainty samples of parameter values consistent with the data. This uncertainty was then propagated through the assessment.

In the application of the parameter estimates for exposure prediction, the estimate of variance about the regression mean ($\sigma^2$) merits particular attention in so far as the estimated value includes the effects of both: (1) the natural (i.e. "true" or actual) variation of *V. vulnificus* densities independent of temperature effects, and (2) the method error attributable to a 3-tube MPN procedure. The natural component of the residual (unexplained) variation represents real variation due to effects other than temperature, such as that associated with variations in salinity and other, as yet unidentified factors. The method error component of the variation is artefactual and an estimate of this must be subtracted from the total residual variation in order to obtain an estimate of the natural variation. For the 3-tube MPN procedure, the method error has been estimated to be 0.12 (DePaola et al., 1997). Consequently, an estimate of the natural (population) variation of $\log_{10}$ *V. vulnificus* per gram (in composites of 12 oysters) was obtained by subtracting 0.12 from the estimated total observed residual variation ($\sigma^2$). For example, the MLE of the total variation is $0.73^2$ based on the Motes et al. data (after averaging replicate measurements per sampling occasion). This estimate corresponds to the mode of the uncertainty distribution of values for this parameter. The corresponding mode of the inferred uncertainty distribution of values for the natural variation is 0.64 (i.e. $0.73^2 - 0.12$) with similar calculations applying to other percentiles of the uncertainty distribution. The same method error was assumed to apply to both the Motes et al. and Tamplin data sets.

Although not incorporated in the present assessment, Motes et al. found that salinity had an appreciable effect on *V. vulnificus* numbers in the Gulf of Mexico. Based on a combined temperature and salinity regression model that is quadratic for both of these factors, Figure 3 illustrates the effect of ignoring salinity and predicting *V. vulnificus* numbers based on the temperature alone for these data. The temperature and salinity regression indicates that optimal salinity for *V. vulnificus* was approximately 17 ppt. For salinities between 12 and 24 ppt, ignoring the effect of salinity will at most over-predict $\log_{10}$ *V. vulnificus*/g by 10% when water temperature is greater than 25°C. However, extremes of salinities, i.e. <10 or >25 ppt, can be detrimental to *V. vulnificus* survival, and predictions of *V. vulnificus* numbers at these extremes based on temperature alone may over-predict by >20% depending upon the temperature. The potential for over-prediction is more pronounced at lower water temperatures.

It should be noted that these predictions assume a continuous (quadratic) effect of salinity on *V. vulnificus* levels. The quadratic model is valid only within a range of salinities about the central (optimal) salinity level. As already indicated, based on comparison of *V. vulnificus* levels observed in high versus moderate salinity regions, there is an apparent abrupt change of the salinity effect at or slightly above 30 ppt. Consequently, the quadratic model of salinity effect can not be used to extrapolate across the apparent discontinuity and the effect of high (>30 ppt) salinity is addressed separately.

### 3.4.1.3. Prediction of the distribution of at-harvest *V. vulnificus* numbers at high (>30 ppt) salinities

While salinities >30 ppt were rarely observed by Motes et al. or Tamplin in Gulf Coast oyster growing waters they were typical of growing areas sampled on the Atlantic coast of the USA (North and South Carolina) (Motes et al., 1998). The *V. vulnificus* levels in most oyster samples were non-detectable when salinity exceeded 30 ppt, regardless of temperature (Table 3). Similar results were obtained from a study in Tokyo Bay in Japan (Table 4) and a recent study in India (Parvathi et al., 2004). This may be an important consideration in countries such as New Zealand that have a major portion of their oyster production in high salinity waters.

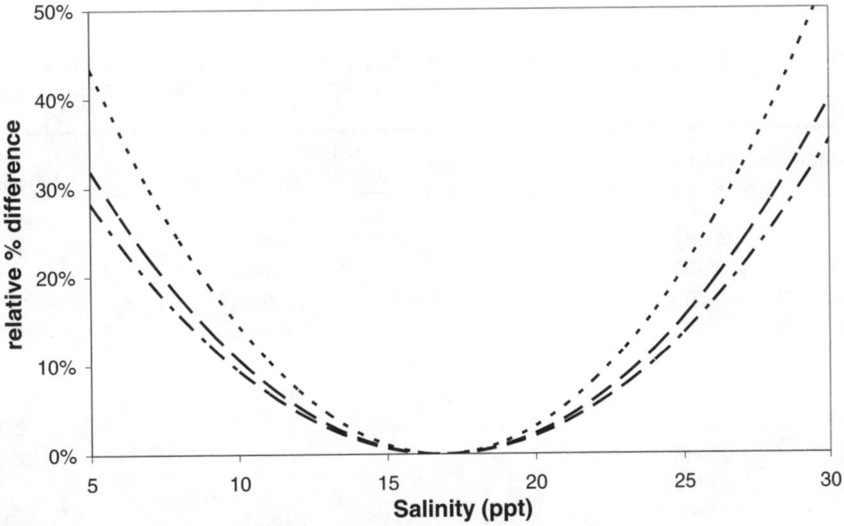


**Figure 3.** Differences in predictions obtained from a temperature-only compared with a temperature and salinity model for $\log_{10}$ *V. vulnificus* in Gulf Coast oysters at harvest. This relationship may not be applicable to other areas or species.

- - - - - - - Relative difference between models at temperatures of 20°C
——— Relative difference between models at temperatures of 25°C
—·—·— Relative difference between models at temperatures of 30°C

**Table 3.** Effect of high (>30 ppt) versus moderate (<30 ppt) salinity on the frequency of detection of *V. vulnificus* and estimates of mean *V. vulnificus*/g in oysters sampled from selected USA Atlantic and Gulf Coast harvest areas (Motes et al., 1998).

| Salinity range | Temperature range | No. of samples | Samples with detectable *V. vulnificus* levels | Mean *V. vulnificus*/g(1) |
|---|---|---|---|---|
| <30 ppt | <20°C | 86 | 62.8% | 140 |
| <30 ppt | 20–25°C | 87 | 90.8% | 1360 |
| <30 ppt | 25–30°C | 157 | 96.2% | 3120 |
| <30 ppt | >30°C | 50 | 96.0% | 3170 |
| <30 ppt | all | 380 | 87.4% | 2050 |
| >30 ppt | < 20°C | 22 | 40.9% | 2.8 |
| >30 ppt | 20–25°C | 33 | 30.3% | 19.5 |
| >30 ppt | 25–30°C | 30 | 23.3% | 2.7 |
| >30 ppt | >30°C | 14 | 35.7% | 4.2 |
| >30 ppt | all | 99 | 31.3% | 8.5 |

NOTES: (1) Mean values calculated by averaging *V. vulnificus*/g (Vv/g) after imputing half the limit of detection (LOD) for samples with <0.3 MPN/g or <3 MPN/g; estimates are likely to be biased high as a consequence of imputing half the limit of detection (LOD) for non-detectable outcomes and failure to correct for the presence of method error.

**Table 4.** Effect of high (>30 ppt) versus moderate (<30 ppt) salinity on the frequency of detection of *V. vulnificus* and estimates of mean *V. vulnificus*/g in oysters sampled from Tokyo Bay, Japan (Oonaka et al., 2002).

| Salinity range | Temperature range | No. of samples | Samples with detectable *V. vulnificus* levels | mean *V. vulnificus*/g(1) |
|---|---|---|---|---|
| <30 ppt | <20°C | 0 | – | – |
| <30 ppt | 20–25°C | 402 | 4.48% | 0.16 |
| <30 ppt | 25–30°C | 749 | 50.20% | 86 |
| <30 ppt | >30°C | 142 | 90.85% | 1116 |
| <30 ppt | all | 1293 | 40.45% | 172 |
| >30 ppt | < 20°C | 43 | 0.00% | 0.15 |
| >30 ppt | 20–25°C | 364 | 8.52% | 0.31 |
| >30 ppt | 25–30°C | 156 | 50.64% | 32.98 |
| >30 ppt | >30°C | 0 | – | – |
| >30 ppt | all | 563 | 19.9% | 9.3 |

NOTES: (1) Mean values calculated by averaging *V. vulnificus*/g (Vv/g) after imputing half the limit of detection (LOD) for samples with <0.3 MPN/g; estimates are likely to be biased high as a consequence of imputing half the limit of detection (LOD) for non-detectable outcomes and failure to correct for the presence of method error.

Unfortunately, the high prevalence of non-detectable levels of *V. vulnificus* severely complicates efforts to quantitatively model effects of temperature and salinity in high salinity regions. Furthermore, given the apparent abrupt change in *V. vulnificus* levels at (or near) 30 ppt, the relationship between *V. vulnificus* levels versus temperature and salinity in high salinity regions can not be inferred from data obtained in moderate (or low) salinity regions. Consequently, the distribution of at-harvest *V. vulnificus* numbers in high salinity regions was not quantitatively modelled. Rather, based on imputing conservative estimates for non-detectable samples, worst case estimates of harvest densities were obtained based on the

Motes et al. and the Tokyo Bay data (Oonaka et al., 2002). The effect of temperature was examined by partitioning the data into temperature ranges. A similar treatment of the data at moderate or low salinity (<30 ppt) is given in Tables 3 and 4 for comparison with the results at >30 ppt.

When salinity was >30 ppt, 69% of USA samples and 80% of Tokyo Bay samples were less than the limit of detection (generally 0.3 MPN/g). Overall, conservative estimates of mean levels at >30 ppt were comparable with estimates of 8.5 and 9.3 *V. vulnificus*/g based on the USA and Japanese data, respectively. No temperature effect was evident in the USA data at high salinity but this was probably a consequence of the relatively small number of samples obtained at high salinity. Based on the Tokyo Bay data, with approximately 500 samples at >30 ppt, there was an apparent trend in both the proportion of samples with detectable *V. vulnificus* and the mean *V. vulnificus*/g across three temperature categories. However, even at the highest temperature category with sample information (25–30°C), mean *V. vulnificus*/g was not substantially greater than 30 MPN/g in Tokyo Bay.

For both the USA and Japanese data, mean *V. vulnificus*/g was consistently higher when salinity was <30 ppt for all temperature ranges but the difference was much more pronounced with the USA data. Part of this difference may be explained by generally higher salinities in Tokyo Bay, even when salinities are <30 ppt. For the <30 ppt salinity category, mean salinity was 24.4 ppt for the Tokyo Bay data compared with 16.8 ppt for the USA data. For the USA data, estimates of mean *V. vulnificus*/g versus the temperature categories given in Table 3 for salinities <30 ppt are consistent with the estimated regression relationship shown in Figure 2.

### 3.4.2. Post-harvest

The numbers of *V. vulnificus* at consumption are influenced by ambient air temperatures at harvest, the time from harvest until the oysters are placed under refrigeration, the time it takes the oysters to cool once under refrigeration, and the length of refrigeration time until consumption. Estimates of post-harvest growth addressed in this section pertain specifically to oysters harvested from moderate or low salinity regions (<30 ppt). These estimates may not be relevant to oysters harvested from high (>30 ppt) salinity areas because oysters harvested from such areas would retain high salinity levels through post-harvest transport and storage and this could substantially reduce post-harvest growth.

#### 3.4.2.1. Growth of *V. vulnificus* from harvest to first refrigeration

The growth model used in the present assessment is the 3-phase linear growth model advocated for microbial risk assessment by Buchanan, Whiting and Damert (1997). This is the same (primary) growth model used in the FAO/WHO-VPRA and the FDA-VPRA. The growth prediction equation of this model is:

$$\log_{10}(N(t)) = \min\{\log_{10}(N(0)) + \mu_m * t, A\}$$

where $N(0)$ denotes the initial number of organisms per g (i.e. at time of harvest), and $N(t)$ denotes the predicted number at t intervals of time (hours) post-harvest. The parameters of the equation are the maximum growth rate ($\mu_m$) and the maximum density ($A$).

A secondary model of microbial growth relating the growth rate to ambient holding temperature is assumed. This secondary model is:

$$\mu_m(T) = \max\{0, \alpha*(T - T_0)\}$$

where $T$ denotes hold temperature and the parameters of the equation are the temperature below which growth does not occur ($T_0$) and the slope ($\alpha$) of a growth rate versus temperature relationship.

Comparative studies of the numbers of *V. vulnificus* in oysters received at processing plants versus oysters at harvest (Ruple and Cook, 1992) and experimental studies with shellstock oysters stored under different temperature regimes clearly indicate that post-harvest multiplication is substantial at ambient air temperatures of ~25°C, which are typical in the USA Gulf Coast in late spring through to early autumn. The best available data to estimate this parameter are provided by two studies (Cook, 1994, 1997a). It is also apparent that the minimum temperature required for growth of *V. vulnificus* is approximately 13°C (Kaspar and Tamplin, 1993). Below this temperature, *V. vulnificus* numbers decrease over time and *V. vulnificus* can enter a viable but non-culturable (VBNC) state (Oliver, 1995).

Figure 4 presents data on the growth of *V. vulnificus* in oysters where oysters were held for up to 14 hours at ambient air temperatures ranging from 24° to 32°C (Cook, 1997a). Table 5 lists the observed growth rates for *V. vulnificus* at various temperatures. A 0.75 $\log_{10}$ increase in numbers was observed over a period of 30 hours when oysters were held at 18°C (Cook, 1994). For oysters harvested during the summer and stored at ambient air temperatures ranging from 24° to 33°C (average 28°C), a 1.3 $\log_{10}$ increase in *V. vulnificus* numbers was observed over 7.5 hours, with a plateau of approximately 2 $\log_{10}$ increase after a period of 14 hours (Cook, 1997a). In an earlier study, oysters stored under refrigeration at 18°C were found to have an average increase of approximately 0.75 $\log_{10}$ over a period of 30 hours (Cook, 1994). Thus, the maximal growth rate is approximately 0.025/hour at 18°C and 0.175/hour at 28°C (for periods of less than 14 hours). Assuming no growth at 13°C, regression of maximal growth rate against temperature gives an estimate of 0.011 $hr^{-1}\,°C^{-1}$ for the slope factor $\alpha$ above the threshold temperature of 13°C (i.e. a linear regression of growth rate versus temperature above 13°C where growth rate is assumed to equal zero at 13°C). The remaining parameter in the primary growth model, the maximum density, was inferred to be equal to $10^6$/g on the basis of several studies that have shown this to be the highest level found in oysters regardless of harvest and post-harvest conditions (Cook, 1994, 1997a; Cook *et al.*, 2002).

Based on the parameter estimates for the primary and secondary growth models, predictions of *V. vulnificus* growth from an initial level of 3 $\log_{10}$ per g are illustrated in Figure 5 for ambient air temperatures of 18°, 20°, 26° and 32°C.

**Table 5.** *V. vulnificus* growth rate versus temperature.

| Study | Holding temperature | Growth rate ($\log_{10}$ per hr) | Assumptions or limitations |
|---|---|---|---|
| Cook, 1997a | 28°C | 0.175 | Ambient air temperature varied from 24 to 33°C, with assumed average of 28°C |
| Cook, 1994 | 18°C | 0.025 | Rate per hour assumed constant with observed average 0.75 $\log_{10}$ increase (n = 5) over 30-hour period |
| Kaspar and Tamplin, 1993 | 13°C | | Presumed no-growth temperature |

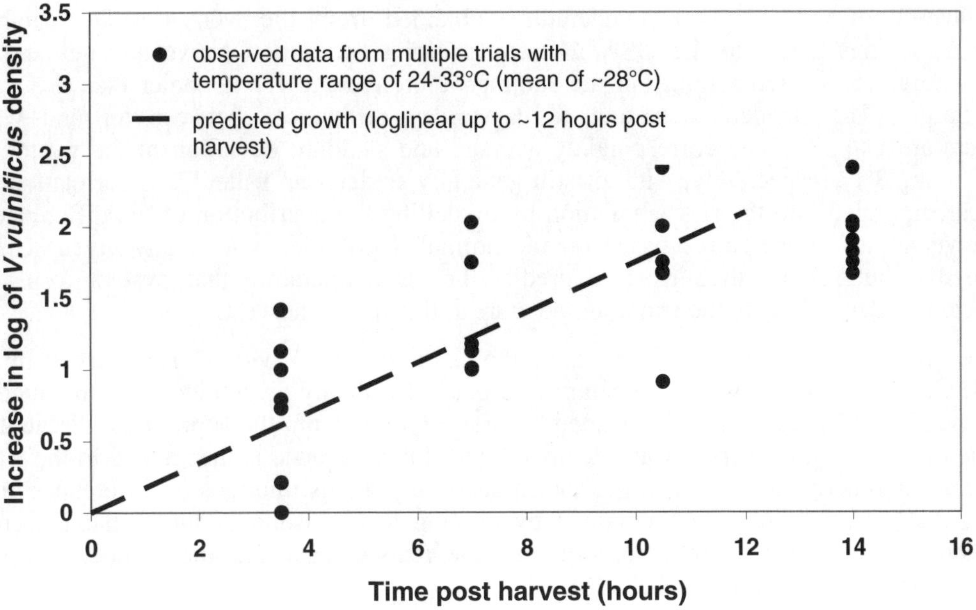


**Figure 4**. Post-harvest growth of *V. vulnificus*.

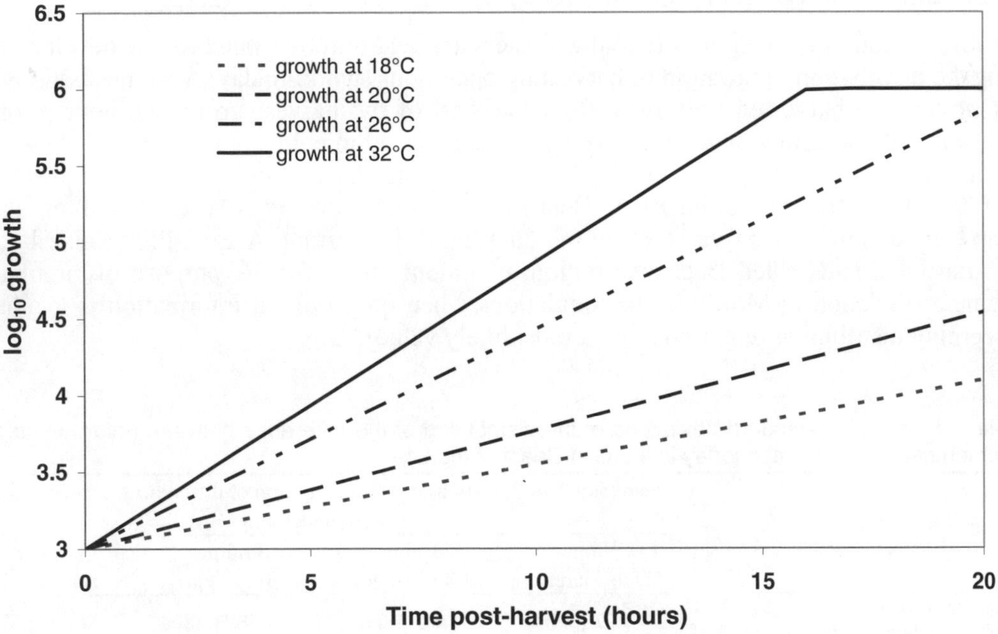


**Figure 5**. Predicted post-harvest growth of *V. vulnificus* from an initial level of 3 $log_{10}$/g.

#### 3.4.2.2. Distribution of ambient air temperature

Examination of water and air temperatures obtained from the NOAA/NBDC database (NOAA, various dates) in the USA indicate a strong correlation between water and air temperature. The air temperature in the summer is on average 1.7°C cooler than the water temperature. The standard deviation of day-to-day differences between air and water temperature is 1.3°C. The corresponding average and standard deviation in the winter are 1.1°C and 3.3°C, respectively, with air still generally cooler than water. This correlation has been incorporated into the risk simulation by modelling the distribution of the difference in water versus air temperatures based on the normal distribution within any given season. These distributions are then used to predict the air temperature that oysters would be subjected to, depending on the water temperature at the time of harvest.

Specifically, in the process of simulating the distribution of *V. vulnificus* at harvest by the Monte Carlo method, the water temperature associated with any given outcome is retained. A corresponding air temperature is obtained by first sampling from the appropriate distribution for the difference in air versus water temperature. This difference is then added to the water temperature to derive a corresponding air temperature. The distributions of differences in air versus water temperature were obtained by pooling the (seasonal) data available from a representative near-shore buoy across all available years of data. The mean and variance of these distributions are shown in Table 6.

This is the same approach to modelling of air temperatures as used in the *V. parahaemolyticus* risk assessment (FDA, 2001; FAO/WHO, in press) and was taken from that work for the purposes of this risk assessment.

#### 3.4.2.3. Distribution of the length of time oysters are left unrefrigerated

The distribution of the length of time that oysters are held unrefrigerated can be developed by using the distribution of duration of harvesting operations (working day), with the assumption that oysters are harvested uniformly from the start of the harvest up to one hour prior to conclusion of harvesting, when they are landed and placed in cold storage. Table 7 shows the minimum, maximum and most likely duration of oyster harvesting estimated for the USA Gulf Coast. In the risk simulation, Beta-PERT distributions were used based on these parameters to simulate the variation in the duration of harvesting. A Beta-PERT distribution is a translated and scaled Beta distribution, commonly used for the purpose of simulating parameter variation in Monte Carlo simulations when only limited information is available concerning distribution (e.g. min., max., most likely value).

**Table 6.** Means and standard deviations of the distribution of the difference between recorded air and water temperatures (°C) at midday in the Gulf Coast of the USA.

| Region (data source) | Mean (standard deviation) of the distribution of differences between air and water temperature | | | |
|---|---|---|---|---|
| | Winter (Jan-March) | Spring (April-June) | Summer (July-Sept) | Autumn (Oct-Dec) |
| Gulf Coast, USA (Dauphin Island, AL buoy) | -1.07 (3.3) | -1.24 (1.63) | -1.66 (1.33) | -1.62 (3.3) |

SOURCE OF DATA: http://www.seaboard.nbdc.noaa.gov/Maps/Wrldmap.shtml

The parameters for these distributions were estimated from data collected during a 1995–1996 FDA Gulf Coast Seafood Laboratory (GCSL) survey in the USA (Cook, 1997b). These data included dealer-reported statistics on the length of harvest. The study was conducted in several Gulf Coast states of the USA during the autumn of two successive years; one season prior to initiation of the NSSP time-to-refrigeration requirements (for states in the USA whose product has been confirmed as the source of two or more *V. vulnificus* illnesses) and then the following year, after implementation. The survey data indicates that the state of Louisiana, with ostensibly more remote harvest areas, has substantially longer harvesting operations than the other Gulf Coast States. Distributions for time unrefrigerated were therefore developed separately for Louisiana versus the other Gulf Coast States. The overall distribution of time unrefrigerated was then obtained as the weighted recombination of these distributions, given that Louisiana accounts for ~50% of the total Gulf Coast harvest. Survey data from Texas were taken to be representative of the harvest practices of the other (non-Louisiana) states.

The duration of harvesting reported in the dealer survey data in 1996, after initiation of the NSSP requirements, was assumed to apply to the spring, summer and autumn seasons. During the winter, when cooler water conditions prevail, the temperatures are generally below the threshold associated with the shorter time-to-refrigeration requirement, so survey data obtained in 1995, prior to implementation of the NSSP, were assumed to apply.

Harvesting of oysters was assumed to occur uniformly from the start of harvest until one hour prior to the end of the harvest operation. The distribution of the duration that the oysters were held unrefrigerated was simulated by first sampling from the distribution for the duration of the harvest operation and then sampling from a uniform distribution with a minimum of one hour and a maximum corresponding to the randomly selected duration of harvest. Because they are harvested over the length of harvesting operations, the mean time that oysters remain unrefrigerated is shorter than the maximum length of duration of harvesting.

Overall, the extent of growth occurring prior to the time of first refrigeration (i.e. time at which the oysters are first placed in refrigerated storage) was simulated by:

- sampling air temperature corresponding to the water temperature at harvest;
- sampling duration of harvest;
- sampling the length of time unrefrigerated given a particular duration of harvest; and
- calculating the extent of growth expected considering both the given duration unrefrigerated and the air temperature.

As with the distribution of ambient air temperature, this is the same distribution as is used in the *V. parahaemolyticus* risk assessment and was taken from that work for the purposes of this risk assessment.

**Table 7.** Minimum, maximum and most likely duration of oyster harvest (length of harvesting operation) for different seasons and subregions of the USA Gulf Coast.

| Location in the USA | Duration of harvest (hours) | | | |
|---|---|---|---|---|
| | Winter (Jan-March) | Spring (April-June) | Summer (July-Sept) | Autumn (Oct-Dec) |
| Gulf Coast - LA (50% of harvest) (pre-NSSP Control plan in LA in winter; others as ICP) | max = 13<br>min = 7<br>most likely = 12 | max = 11<br>min = 5<br>most likely = 9 | max = 11<br>min = 5<br>most likely = 9 | max = 13<br>min = 7<br>most likely = 12 |
| Gulf Coast - FL, AL, TX (50% of harvest) (assumed same as pre-NSSP ICP in Gulf-TX in winter; NSSP Control otherwise) | max = 11<br>min = 2<br>most likely = 8 | max = 10<br>min = 3<br>most likely = 7 | max = 10<br>min = 3<br>most likely = 7 | max = 10<br>min = 3<br>most likely = 7 |

KEY TO STATES: LA = Louisiana; AL = Alabama; TX = Texas; FL = Florida.
SOURCE: Cook, 1997b.

### 3.4.2.4. Growth of *V. vulnificus* during cooling

The time it takes for oysters to cool once under refrigeration is assumed to vary according to the efficiency of the chilling medium, the quantity of oysters to be cooled and their arrangement in the cold room. Data on cooling rates of commercial oyster shellstock was not available. In the USA preliminary GCSL experiments with a single in-shell oyster at 30°C, in which a temperature probe was inserted into its tissue, indicated a cooling rate of approximately 0.5°C/min when placed into a 3°C cooler (A. DePaola, personal communication, 2002). However, 24 oysters in an uninsulated plastic container required approximately 7 hours to cool from 26°C to 3°C. These data suggest considerable uncertainty for cooling times after oysters are refrigerated and it was concluded that a uniform distribution between 1 and 10 hours would be appropriate to describe the current state of knowledge, with all values in this range being equally likely regardless of initial air temperature (i.e. temperature difference).

At the start of the cooling period, when oysters are first placed under refrigeration, the growth rate was taken to be equal to the initial rate as determined by ambient air temperature. At the end of the cooling period, when oysters have reached storage temperatures, it was assumed that there is no further growth and that numbers will decline slowly thereafter. Implicitly, this assumes that there is no appreciable temperature abuse after oysters have been placed in cold storage. As the rate at which oysters cool during cold storage is not known, it was assumed that during the period of cooling, the growth rate of *V. vulnificus* decreases uniformly to zero. Once again, model assumptions for growth during the process of cooling were the same as those used in the *V. parahaemolyticus* risk assessment.

### 3.4.2.5. Die-off of *V. vulnificus* during cold storage

*V. vulnificus* is more susceptible to cold than *V. parahaemolyticus*. Based on ISSC/FDA retail data (Cook et al., 2002), it has been estimated that *V. vulnificus* numbers decline by 0.041 logs per day under normal conditions of cold storage in the USA marketplace. Minimum, maximum and most likely duration of storage of oyster lots sampled in this same study were used in the FAO/WHO-VPRA to define a distribution of storage times for the USA marketplace. The same distribution was assumed here.

Data from a retail study for the time between harvest and sample collection were assumed to be a reliable estimate for the refrigerated storage time prior to consumption. Summary statistics on the storage time for samples obtained during the study are shown in Table 8. A small degree of error may be introduced by assuming that these data are representative of storage time insofar as samples were generally collected on a Monday or a Tuesday and most servings are consumed in restaurants during weekends. Since this was a year-long nationwide survey, the mean of 7.7 days and range of 1–21 days were assumed to be representative of all seasons. In the simulation, a Beta-PERT distribution based on the minimum, maximum and mode (most likely value) was used in order to obtain a smooth representation of the variation in the duration of storage time. Refrigerated storage time can vary significantly from one country to another. For example, in Japan the mean is 1 day, with a range of 0.125 to 1.04 days. In Australia it can range from 1 to 10 days, with a most likely time of 6 days, while in New Zealand, storage time tends to be shorter, between 1 and 5 days with a most likely time of 2 days (FAO/WHO, in press).

## 3.5. Simulation results

Monte Carlo simulations of the distribution of *V. vulnificus* at harvest and at selected points in the production-consumption process continuum were obtained using the simulation program Analytica® (Analytica, Lumina Decision Systems, Inc., USA). As outlined in the discussion above, the output distributions were based primarily on water temperature, the derived regression relationship between $\log_{10}$ *V. vulnificus* numbers and water temperature, *V. vulnificus* growth rate versus temperature and various distribution parameters, which affect the extent of microbial growth and survival post-harvest.

Seasonal *V. vulnificus* exposure associated with USA Gulf Coast oysters was simulated. Parameter distributions were obtained by the Monte Carlo method using a sample size of 10 000. The effect of year-to-year variation in mean and variance of water temperature distributions was evaluated based on 100 Monte Carlo samples of water temperature parameters (i.e. mean and variance). Using the selected Motes et al. data with the two replicates averaged, statistical summaries of the parameter distributions obtained by Monte Carlo sampling, averaged over the year-to-year variations in water temperature, are shown in Table 9.

**Table 8.** Summary statistics of the distribution of storage times (time under refrigeration in days) of oysters samples collected during a retail study.

| Storage Time (days) | Consumed locally (within the same region of harvest) | Non-local (transported outside region of harvest) | Overall |
|---|---|---|---|
| Minimum | 1 | 2 | 1 |
| Maximum | 20 | 21 | 21 |
| Mean | 6.3 | 9.9 | 7.7 |
| Most likely | 6 | 5 | 6 |

SOURCE OF DATA: Cook *et al.*, 2002.

**Table 9**. Summary output of the simulation of environmental parameters, oyster handling conditions, *V. vulnificus* growth, survival and numbers from harvest to consumption in USA Gulf Coast oysters in the winter (January - March), spring (April – June), summer (July – September) and autumn (October - December).

| Distribution Parameter | Winter (January - March) | Spring (April – June) | Summer (July – September) | Autumn (October - December) |
|---|---|---|---|---|
| | Mean (standard deviation)[1] | | | |
| Water temperature (°C) | 14.2 (2.7) | 24.5 (3.5) | 28.9 (1.5) | 17.9 (4.5) |
| $Log_{10}$ *V. vulnificus*/g at harvest | 0.47 (1.09) | 2.75 (0.82) | 3.27 (0.64) | 1.39 (1.36) |
| *V. vulnificus*/g at harvest | 40 | 2 600 | 5 600 | 500 |
| Air-water temperature difference (°C) | -1.07 (3.3) | -1.24 (1.63) | -1.66 (1.33) | -1.62 (3.3) |
| Air temperature (°C) | 13.1 (4.3) | 23.3 (4.1) | 27.2 (2.0) | 16.4 (5.5) |
| Time on the water | 9.4 hours | 7.7 hours | 7.7 hours | 9.1 hours |
| Time oysters unrefrigerated | 5.2 hours | 4.4 hours | 4.4 hours | 5.0 hours |
| $Log_{10}$ growth prior to refrigeration | 0.11 (0.18) | 0.49 (0.32) | 0.68 (0.35) | 0.24 (0.30) |
| $Log_{10}$ growth during cool down | 0.06 (0.10) | 0.37 (0.21) | 0.50 (0.22) | 0.15 (0.18) |
| Die-off during storage (in logs) | 0.31 | 0.31 | 0.31 | 0.31 |
| $Log_{10}$ *V. vulnificus*/g at consumption | 0.30 (1.22) | 3.28 (1.08) | 4.15 (0.78) | 1.45 (1.64) |
| *V. vulnificus*/g at consumption | 80 | 21 400 | 57 000 | 3 700 |
| Oysters per serving | 13.7 | 13.7 | 13.7 | 13.7 |
| Grams per serving | 196 | 196 | 196 | 196 |
| Total *V. vulnificus* ingested per serving | $1.6 \times 10^4$ | $4.2 \times 10^6$ | $1.1 \times 10^7$ | $7.3 \times 10^5$ |

NOTES: (1) For distributions that are approximately normally distributed, the standard deviation is given in parentheses; no standard deviation is tabulated for those distributions that are highly skewed. For skewed distributions (*V. vulnificus*/g), the median of the uncertainty distribution of mean *V. vulnificus*/g is given.

Overall, the simulation results suggest that *V. vulnificus* numbers increase post-harvest an average of 0.90 $log_{10}$ MPN/g during the summer harvest season and decrease an average of 0.20 $log_{10}$ MPN/g during the winter harvest season. Variation in water and air temperatures and the characteristics of harvesting duration and storage time have the effect of increasing the variation of *V. vulnificus* numbers at each point along the harvest-to-consumption continuum. For the USA Gulf Coast winter, the standard deviation of *V. vulnificus* numbers (in 12-oyster composites) is 1.22 $log_{10}$ at consumption compared with 1.09 $log_{10}$ at harvest. Due to the positive skew of the distributions, the mean density of *V. vulnificus* per gram is greater than the antilog of mean $log_{10}$ MPN per gram. Mean densities of 57 000 and 80 per gram were obtained for the summer and winter harvest seasons, respectively. Given an average serving size of 196 grams of oyster meat weight (Cook *et al.*, 2002; A. DePaola, personal communication 2002) these average numbers correspond to average ingested doses of $1.1 \times 10^7$ and $1.6 \times 10^4$ respectively.

Representative outputs of the simulation are shown in Figures 6 to 8. These graphs illustrate the effect of post-harvest parameters on the location and shape of the distribution of *V. vulnificus* per gram. Generally, each stage of the harvest to consumption continuum shifts the mean $log_{10}$ numbers per gram, with a concomitant increase in the variability about the mean from one sample of oysters to the next.

Figure 6 shows typical distributions of the water and air temperature obtained for the Gulf Coast summer. These distributions are normal by assumption. As evident in the figure, the distribution of air temperature has a mean that is slightly less than that of water and exhibits more variation (i.e. spread). The variation in temperatures drives numbers at harvest and determines variability in extent of growth occurring after harvest. Together with parameters affecting harvest duration (e.g. distribution of time prior to first refrigeration as shown in Figure 7), the growth rate of *V. vulnificus* post-harvest and survival during storage is used to derive the distribution of numbers at the time of consumption. The difference in *V. vulnificus* numbers at harvest versus at consumption is shown is Figure 8. The *V. vulnificus* numbers at consumption are slightly less than 1 $\log_{10}$ higher than those at harvest during the relatively higher-risk summer season.

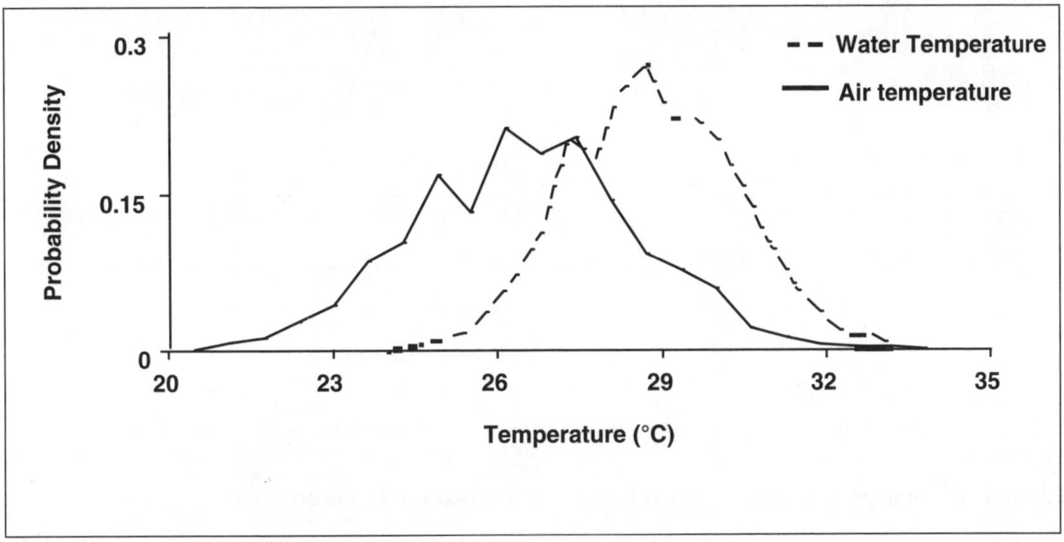


**Figure 6.** Distribution of typical day-to-day "noontime" water and air temperatures for the USA Gulf Coast summer.

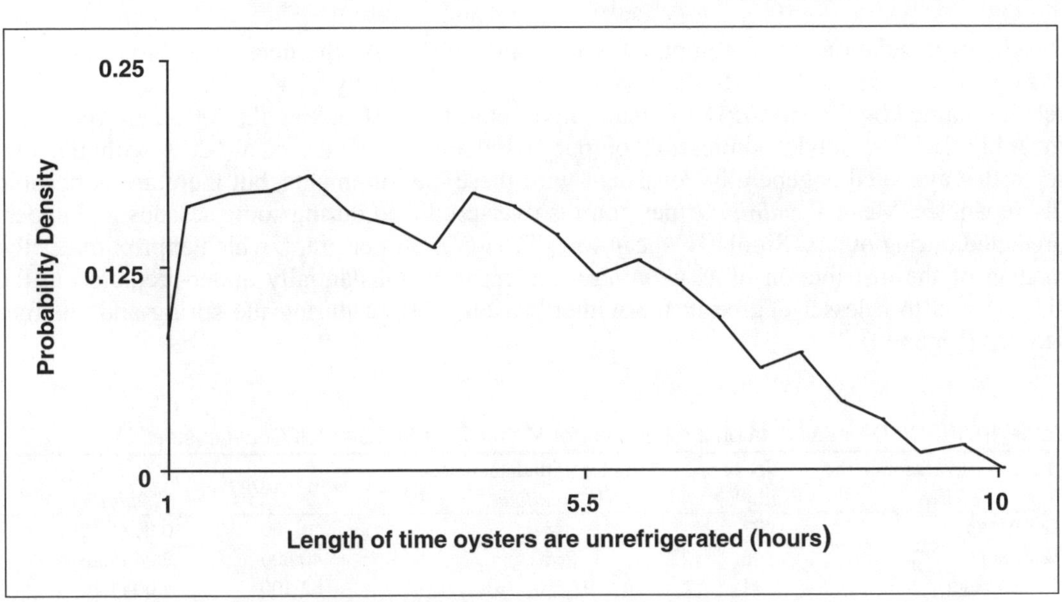


**Figure 7**. Distribution of the time that oysters are held unrefrigerated post-harvest.

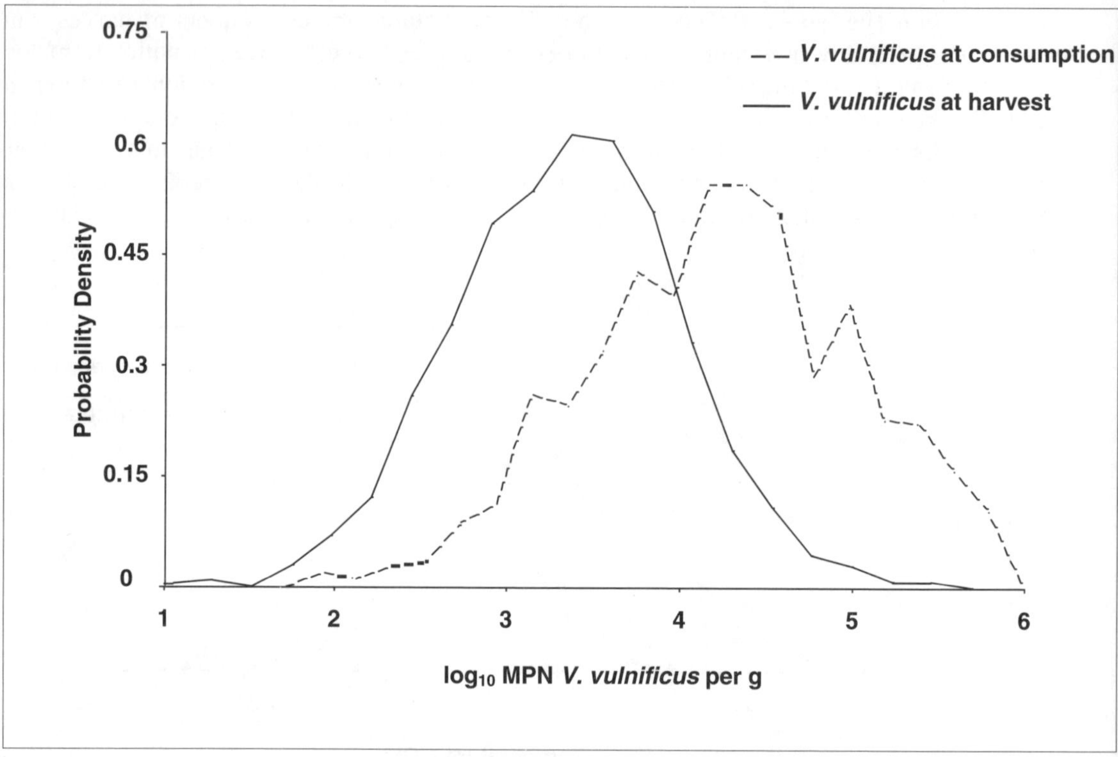


**Figure 8.** Distribution of *V. vulnificus* (Vv) numbers at harvest versus consumption.

## 3.6. Model validation

Results of simulations were compared with available data on the density of *V. vulnificus* in oysters at retail in the USA. Summary statistics for the density of *V. vulnificus* in oysters at retail, obtained by the ISSC/FDA collaborative retail study (Cook et al., 2002), are presented in Table 10. The model simulation output based on the Motes et al. data with the two replicates averaged is generally consistent with these measurements, but there are noticeable discrepancies. Mean *V. vulnificus* per gram is over-predicted during some seasons and under-predicted during others. Similarly, mean $\log_{10}$ *V. vulnificus* per gram, which approximates the median of the distribution of *V. vulnificus* per gram, is substantially under-predicted in the autumn and to a lesser degree in the winter season, but not during the spring and summer seasons (Figure 9).

**Table 10.** ISSC/FDA retail data on the numbers of *V. vulnificus* in USA Gulf Coast oysters.

| Region and season in the USA | No. of samples | Samples with detectable *V. vulnificus* | *V. vulnificus*/g$^{(1)}$ | $\log_{10}$ *V. vulnificus*/g$^{(2)}$ |
|---|---|---|---|---|
| Gulf/winter | 37 | 84% | 60 | 0.60 (1.12) |
| Gulf/spring | 46 | 96% | 40 800 | 3.24 (1.28) |
| Gulf/summer | 41 | 97.5% | 62 100 | 4.00 (1.16) |
| Gulf/autumn | 46 | 96% | 10 700 | 3.08 (1.48) |

NOTE: (1) Arithmetic mean. (2) Mean and standard deviation.

The differences between observed versus predicted mean $\log_{10}$ *V. vulnificus* per gram appear to be largely a consequence of warmer than normal water (and air) temperatures that were occurring in the USA Gulf Coast from September 1998 to March 1999 due to a La Nina weather pattern. As will be discussed further in later sections of this document, substituting the autumn-1998-specific and winter-1999-specific temperature data in the simulation reduces much of the discrepancy in predicted versus observed mean $\log_{10}$ *V. vulnificus* per gram (Figure 9). Differences in observed versus predicted mean *V. vulnificus* per gram are more problematic. To the extent that *V. vulnificus* per gram is approximately lognormal, the mean of the distribution of *V. vulnificus* per gram is a function of both the mean and standard deviation of the distribution of $\log_{10}$ *V. vulnificus* per gram. Thus, over-prediction of mean *V. vulnificus* per gram by the model simulation could be due to over-prediction of either the mean or the standard deviation of $\log_{10}$ *V. vulnificus* per gram.

Since, after correcting for temperature, differences in predicted versus observed mean $\log_{10}$ *V. vulnificus* per gram are not large (Figure 9), it appears more likely that differences in observed versus predicted mean *V. vulnificus* per gram are attributable to over-prediction of the population standard deviation of $\log_{10}$ *V. vulnificus* per gram. Here it is relevant to note that the standard deviation of observed $\log_{10}$ *V. vulnificus* per gram shown in Table 10 is likely to be inflated by the presence of method error.

The ISSC/FDA retail study (Cook et al., 2002) employed an MPN procedure for enumeration and thus a percentage of the variance of observed $\log_{10}$ numbers is attributable to method error over and above true variation in numbers from one sample to the next. This method error is symmetric and unbiased on the $\log_{10}$ scale but not on the untransformed scale (i.e. MPN or count per gram). The magnitude of this method error is not known precisely since a modified MPN procedure was employed to compensate for the effect of interference observed in the MPN series for these data. Thus, method error could not be estimated and its effect subtracted from the estimates shown in Table 10. The effect of not correcting the estimates for the presence of this method error introduces an upward bias in the estimates of mean *V. vulnificus* per gram. In the model simulation, the error associated with measurements of *V. vulnificus* has already been subtracted out and, consequently, the over-prediction of mean *V. vulnificus* per gram in some seasons may be even greater than that suggested by a simple comparison of the numbers shown in Tables 9 and 10.

Table 11 compares mean *V. vulnificus*/g observed in the ISSC/FDA (Cook et al., 2002) retail study with predicted values at consumption using both average seasonal temperatures and temperature specific to the autumn of 1998 and the winter of 1999 based on the Motes et al. (replicates averaged) and Tamplin data alone and with the pooled data sets. The highest predicted *V. vulnificus* levels for all seasons were obtained based on the Tamplin data and the lowest with the Motes et al. data. The *V. vulnificus* levels observed in the ISSC retail study were considerably lower than any of the predicted values for the autumn of 1998 and the winter of 1999; the Tamplin data over-predicted by a factor of approximately 3 and 20 for the autumn and winter, respectively. Overall, the predictions based on the Motes et al. data were in closest agreement with the retail data but it under-predicted in the spring by a factor of ~2 and over-predicted in the winter by a factor of ~6.5. The estimate of population standard deviation at time of harvest is particularly important, since this is the largest component of the variance in $\log_{10}$ *V. vulnificus* levels at the time of consumption. It is possible that the estimates obtained from analysis of the Motes et al. and Tamplin data are overestimates of the true variation. As discussed in Appendix B and D, there was substantially higher variance in *V. vulnificus* levels observed in the Tamplin study compared with that observed in the Motes et al. study. This may be a consequence of the fact that the studies were undertaken in different periods, locations or that different protocols were used to ensure that no post-harvest growth occurred in collected samples. It is also possible that the true variation in *V. vulnificus* levels changes with season and this is not reflected in the parameter estimates that were obtained from the regression analysis of the harvest density data.

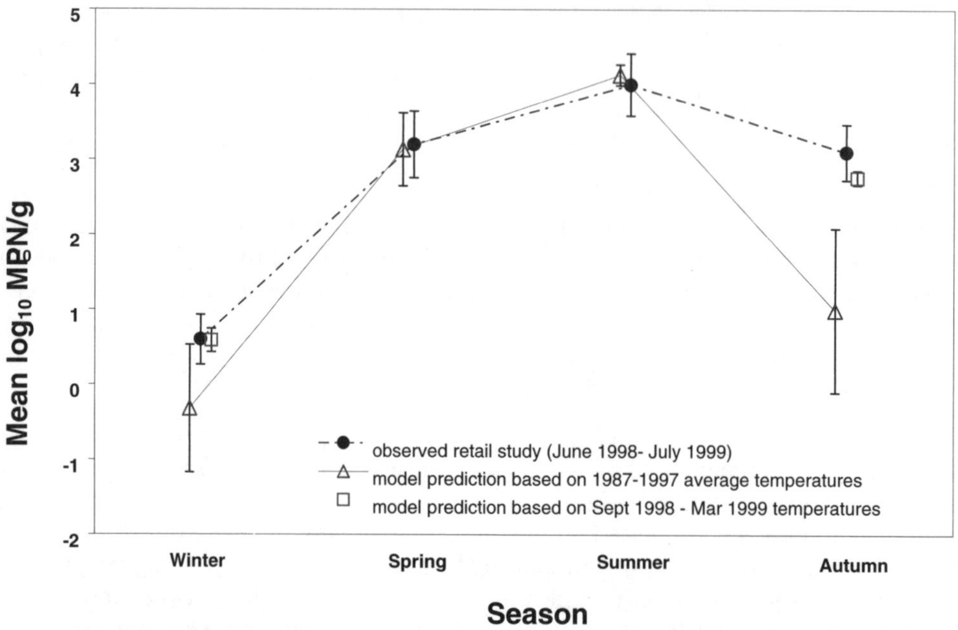


**Figure 9.** Predicted versus observed *V. vulnificus* numbers in retail shell oysters. The error bars denote the 95% confidence intervals for mean $\log_{10}$ levels with respect to the retail data and corresponding uncertainty intervals of the predictions based on model simulations. Best estimates of model-based predictions were taken to be equal to the medians of the respective uncertainty distributions.

**Table 11**. ISSC/FDA retail data (Cook et al., 2002) on the numbers of *V. vulnificus* in USA Gulf Coast oysters compared with alternative model-predicted numbers at consumption derived from different data sets for levels at harvest.

| Region/ Season in USA | Mean *V. vulnificus*/g based on retail data | Mean *V. vulnificus*/g (based on Motes data model)(1) | Mean *V. vulnificus*/g (based on Tamplin data model)(1) | Mean *V. vulnificus*/g (based on pooled data model)(1) |
|---|---|---|---|---|
| Gulf/winter (typical) | – | 80 (20, 610) | 240 (30, 1 800) | 140 (20, 1 000) |
| Gulf/spring (typical) | 40 800 | 21 400 (12 700, 33 500) | 55 300 (21 800, 92 100) | 36 600 (24 100, 55 800) |
| Gulf/summer (typical) | 62 100 | 57 000 (37 900, 70 500) | 131 800 (63 100, 203 000) | 93 400 (72 900, 107 000) |
| Gulf/autumn (typical) | – | 3 700 (1 500, 11 700) | 9 200 (3 300, 25 600) | 6 100 (2 700, 16 500) |
| Gulf/autumn 1998 | 10 700 | 16 100 (11 800, 19 800) | 36 600 (16 600, 59 800) | 25 400 (21 100, 28 800) |
| Gulf/winter 1999 | 60 | 390 (240, 590) | 1 100 (400, 2 200) | 670 (420, 1 000) |

NOTES: (1) median of the uncertainty distribution of model-based simulations and the central 90% interval of the uncertainty distribution (5 and 95 percentiles).

# 4. Hazard characterization

## 4.1. Description of the factors that influence the disease outcome

### 4.1.1. Characteristics of the pathogen

*V. vulnificus* potentially causes mild to moderate gastroenteritis in healthy people who consume contaminated food; however, for a specific subpopulation of susceptible people, *V. vulnificus* can cause a serious septicaemia that frequently leads to death.

#### 4.1.1.1. Genetic factors, such as virulence factors

The virulence factors associated with *V. vulnificus* are poorly characterized. Factors like cytolysin, protease/elastase and phospholipase all may play a role, but none appears to be essential for virulence, as some mutant strains with these factors deleted do not appear to exhibit decreased virulence in animal models (Strom and Paranjpye, 2000). The presence of a capsule appears to be correlated with virulence, but most freshly isolated environmental strains appear to have a capsule, irrespective of their virulence (Strom and Paranjpye, 2000). The virulence factors associated with *V. vulnificus* include a capsule, cytolysin, protease/elastase and phospholipase, but these are found in nearly all clinical and environmental strains (Strom and Paranjpye, 2000). More recent studies (Nilsson et al., 2003) indicate that an rRNA gene sequence may be related to virulence, as the type B sequence was more prevalent in clinical strains (approximately 80%) than in strains isolated from market oysters (approximately 8%). While rRNA type may be a potential virulence marker, the seasonal and regional distribution of rRNA type has not been investigated. Virulence appears to be multifaceted and is not well understood, and therefore, in this risk assessment, all strains were considered virulent.

### 4.1.2. Characteristics of the host

#### 4.1.2.1. Immune and physiological status of the host

Foodborne *V. vulnificus* infection is clearly associated with underlying medical conditions (Strom and Paranjpye, 2000). Liver disease is a prominent risk factor for *V. vulnificus* infection, including cirrhosis due to alcohol consumption. Additional risk factors include diabetes, gastrointestinal disorders (surgery, ulcers), haematological conditions, and immunodeficiency due to underlying conditions such as cancer and treatment of chronic conditions with immunosuppressive agents (arthritis, etc.). As with many other micro-organisms, the pathogenicity of *V. vulnificus* appears to be associated with the availability of free iron in the host (Wright et al., 1981). Many of the known predisposing conditions for infection, particularly chronic liver diseases, are associated with impaired iron metabolism. *V. vulnificus* may pose a small risk to otherwise "healthy" individuals since a small fraction of cases (<5%) occur in individuals without any identifiable risk factor.

*Normal population*

The normal population may be susceptible to a relatively mild gastroenteritis from consumption of seafood's harbouring *V. vulnificus*, but this rarely leads to primary septicaemia (Strom and Paranjpye, 2000). Hence, healthy individuals will be excluded from this assessment, as the focus is the more serious primary septicaemia cases.

*Susceptible population*

The prevalence of predisposing conditions among the adult population (>18 years of age) in the USA has been estimated in a 1997 memorandum to the FDA Office of Seafood Director (Klontz, 1997). These estimates are presented in Table 12.

Using a median value for the prevalence of hepatitis and lupus, these numbers suggest that approximately 7% of the USA adult population is susceptible to infection. Given the uncertainty in prevalence of liver disease (including hepatitis), this number could be as high as ~16%. However, the median estimate of prevalence of liver disease is consistent with results of the 1988 Florida behavioural survey in which 2.4% of raw oyster consumers surveyed reported that they were aware that they had a liver disease (Hlady, Mullen and Hopkin, 1993). Consequently, although it can not be ruled out that up to ~8% of the population have undiagnosed chronic liver conditions, a figure of 7% appears to be a more reasonable estimate of the susceptible population. This represents a population of 13 million individuals in the USA at "high risk" of infection. However, it must be noted that this could be different for other countries and regions, particularly where large numbers of the population suffer from hepatitis.

The overall estimate of size of the susceptible population is somewhat imprecise due to varying case definitions of the disease conditions. For most disease conditions, the estimates presented in Table 12 (Klontz, 1997) are based on cases defined by relatively severe progression (e.g. long-term corticosteroid treatment, end-stage renal disease, etc.). The

**Table 12.** Prevalence rates of *V. vulnificus* risk factors per 100 000 individuals assuming a total USA adult population of 185 000 000 individuals (Klontz, 1997).

| Risk factor | Prevalence per 100 000 individuals |
|---|---|
| Diabetes (insulin-dependent) | 540.5 |
| Liver disease (cirrhosis) | 2000 (range: 1600–9900) |
| Gastric acidity | 38.9 |
| Cancer | 1420.0 |
| Hepatitis (B and C) | (range: 400–1600) |
| Kidney disease | 108.0 |
| Haemochromatosis | 1081.1 |
| AIDS | 540.5 |
| Immune-compromised due to treatment/surgery | |
| Asthma | 25.7 |
| Rheumatoid arthritis | 51.4 |
| Psoriatic arthritis | 37.9 |
| Lupus | (range: 4–250) |
| Polymylagia rheumatica | 53.0 |
| Giant cell arthritis | 12.0 |
| Transplant recipients | 59.5 |
| Total | ~7000 (7%) |

relative risks of infection associated with the identified disease conditions have not been well characterized. There may be a distribution of susceptibility related to progression of each of the various predisposing conditions. For this assessment, relative risks have been assumed to be the same across these identified disease conditions, namely all susceptible individuals are equally susceptible.

#### 4.1.2.2. Age, sex and ethnic group

The vehicle of infection under consideration in this risk assessment for *V. vulnificus* is raw oysters. The consumption patterns for raw oysters in the USA have been estimated for age, sex and ethnic group (Desenclos *et al.*, 1991; Klontz et al., 1995; Timbo *et al.*, 1996; and Flattery and Bashin, 2004). Women comprise only about 10% of reported *V. vulnificus* infections (M. Glatzer, personal communication, 2001). While women consume raw oysters less frequently than men (Flattery and Bashin, 2004), this does not account for the reported magnitude of differences in illness rates. It is not known whether women who consume oysters have different rates of risk factors or some additional protection compared with men.

#### 4.1.2.3. Health behaviours

All *Vibrio* spp. are relatively susceptible to inactivation by cooking. Most of the risk associated with the relevant strains of *Vibrio* spp. in food comes from the consumption of raw oysters or from cross-contamination of other foods by raw seafood or contaminated water. Health behaviours leading to impaired liver function as the result of long-term heavy alcohol consumption are a major risk factor for septicaemia from *V. vulnificus* infection (Klontz, 1997).

#### 4.1.2.4. Genetic factors

Host genetic factors related to susceptibility to *V. vulnificus* gastrointestinal infections are unknown, however, there are many genetic factors associated with the likelihood of the infection to proceed to septicaemia. The presence of a human genetic mutation leading to reduced levels of transferrin, such as hereditary haemochromatosis, results in increased likelihood of septicaemia for the infected individual.

### 4.1.3. Characteristics of the food matrix

#### 4.1.3.1. Fat and salt content

Fat and salt content are probably not relevant in the determination of risk with respect to *Vibrio* spp. While the fat content of a matrix may be relevant with respect to the increase of effective dose of pathogens through protection of *Vibrio* spp. in micelles during gastric passage, there is insufficient evidence to model the degree of increased survival.

#### 4.1.3.2. pH and water activity

*Vibrio* spp. appear to be relatively sensitive to both low pH and dehydration. Because of the nature of most foods associated with the unintended consumption of *Vibrio* spp., pH and water activity are probably not relevant in modelling survival of *V. vulnificus* in raw oysters, although these parameters may be relevant in modelling the growth of *Vibrio* spp. in other foods as a result of cross-contamination.

## 4.2. Public health outcomes

There are numerous reports of sporadic foodborne cases of illness caused by *V. vulnificus,* but outbreaks of illness due to *V. vulnificus* have not to date been associated with consumption of food (Shapiro et al., 1998). An outbreak of wound infections caused by a single clone, designated biogroup 3, was reported among fish handlers in Israel, but there have not been subsequent reports of outbreaks (Bisharat and Raz, 1997).

### 4.2.1. Manifestations of disease

*V. vulnificus* causes mild to severe gastrointestinal illness, potentially progressing to septicaemia, with a significant mortality rate among susceptible populations.

### 4.2.2. Rationale for the biological end points modelled

Septicaemia was the endpoint modelled in this risk assessment, as patients typically present to healthcare systems with this symptom. Based on the available data, this risk assessment considers only reported cases in which a history of consumption of raw Gulf Coast oysters is documented. Because of the severity of the septicaemia, under-reporting was not considered to be substantial (2:1) compared to gastrointestinal illnesses, such as is caused by *V. parahaemolyticus*, which the Centers for Disease Control (CDC) estimates to have a 20:1 under-reporting ratio in the USA (Mead et al., 1999). Additional sources of under-reporting of *V. vulnificus* septicaemia have been suggested, e.g. non routine use of Thiosulfate Citrate Bile Sucrose (TCBS) agar in analysis of samples from non-hospitalized patients (J. Painter, personal communication, 2004).

Data collected by FDA was used in this assessment. Historically, FDA has recorded cases only where patients admitted eating oysters. Patients who ate oysters may have denied oyster consumption, may not have been willing to answer questions, or may have deceased before a food history could be obtained. Alternatively, the number of oyster-associated infections could be estimated from those that did respond to the questionnaire. Another source of under-reporting is the failure to capture all the cases in different reporting systems. Since 1998, most state health departments voluntarily report *V. vulnificus* infections to the CDC Cholera and other Vibrios Surveillance System (COVISS). COVISS is the source of case reports referenced in this risk assessment. However, states may also choose to report to the National Notifiable Diseases Surveillance System (NNDSS). In a recent comparison of both surveillance systems, CDC found that approximately 80% of *V. vulnificus* cases were in common and approximately 20% of cases reported to one system were not reported to the other. Applying the capture-recapture method indicated that multiplying the total number of reported cases to COVISS by 1.25 (1/80%) would be appropriate for estimating the total number of reported cases. Applying the above adjustments would indicate that there are 2.5 times more *V. vulnificus* septicaemia cases associated with raw Gulf Coast oysters than the mean of 32 reported cases from 1995 to 2001. It is possible to make adjustments to account for any possible under-reporting. Although no such adjustments were undertaken in the current risk assessment, it involves shifting the dose-response relationship toward greater risk at a given dose which in turn would lead to an increase in the illness reduction predictions from interventions by a factor of 2.5. For example, a mitigation targeted at reducing *V. vulnificus* to one reported case per year based on this risk assessment, would if adjusted for under-reporting compare to 2.5 annual cases: however while the current risk assessment predicts the number of illnesses prevented to be 31, adjusting for under-reporting would lead to a prediction of 77.5 (31× 2.5) illnesses prevented.

## 4.3. Dose-response relationship

### 4.3.1. Summary of available data

#### 4.3.1.1. Probability of illness given exposure.

There are no human volunteer studies using *V. vulnificus* with which to estimate a dose-response relationship. The available data allows estimation of the relationship by comparing monthly exposure estimates for sensitive populations with monthly observed epidemiological data in the USA in a manner similar to that proposed by Buchanan et al. (1997). A consistent *V. vulnificus* reporting system has been in effect since 1995 in the USA, and CDC data is currently available up to and including 2001.

#### 4.3.1.2. Probability of sequelae given illness and secondary and tertiary transmission

There are no known sequelae associated with *V. vulnificus* septicaemia. There are few, if any, reports of secondary or tertiary transmissions of illnesses caused by *V. vulnificus*.

#### 4.3.1.3. Probability of death given illness

For *V. vulnificus* in the USA, mortality rates are between 50% and 60% for patients with septicaemia (Hlady and Klontz, 1996; Shapiro *et al.*, 1998).

### 4.3.2. Sources of data used

Modelling of the dose-response relationship for *V. vulnificus* was based on estimates of exposure per eating occasion, number of eating occasions in the susceptible population, and month- and year-specific data on the number of oyster-associated cases reported to the USA CDC from 1995 to 2001, as shown in Appendix C. Both the Beta-Poisson and the Exponential model were fitted to the data and the uncertainty of the Beta-Poisson dose-response fit was characterized by considering uncertainty or variability in the number of cases likely to occur at any given exposure and the uncertainty of the mean $\log_{10}$ density of *V. vulnificus* at harvest predicted to be associated with month- and year-specific water temperatures in the Gulf of Mexico.

Typical calculations of mean *V. vulnificus* dose per serving and USA CDC statistics for average number of cases per month are shown in Table 13. The mean *V. vulnificus* numbers in oyster tissue at harvest were obtained by combining data for the USA Gulf Coast water temperatures with the *V. vulnificus* density versus water temperature regression relationship presented in the exposure assessment.

The mean *V. vulnificus* levels at retail were developed in the exposure assessment based on post-harvest handling assumptions, as reported in Section 3, together with estimates of *V. vulnificus*-specific growth rate post-harvest and survival during cold storage. The same methods outlined in the exposure assessment were used here to estimate monthly mean *V. vulnificus* densities at retail. While the estimates shown in Table 13 are typical averages, examination of the water temperature and case series data suggested the potential for year-to-year differences in water temperature affecting illness rates. Consequently, month- and year-specific data were used to develop the dose-response assessment, and the numbers shown in Table 13 are simply intended to be illustrative of the type of calculations that were employed.

The number of servings per month was estimated assuming that 50% of the average landings for that month are consumed raw and then converting to the corresponding number of meals based on average oyster weight and typical number of oysters per serving. While there were some year-to-year differences in aggregate monthly oyster landings, these differences were not substantial compared with the potential effects of water temperature. Consequently, average monthly landing statistics, as shown in Table 13, were used for all years (1995–2001). The number of meals consumed by the susceptible population was estimated as being 7% of total meals. For the purpose of dose-response modelling, the average ingested *V. vulnificus* dose per serving was considered more pertinent than the median (Crump, 1998). The mean is the more pertinent summary statistic in this context as it has been observed that it is the illness burden that is the public health impact of foremost concern and this is in turn determined by the mean (and not necessarily the median) risk per serving in respect to any given collection of (variable) exposures for which illness burden is of interest (see Appendix C). Thus an estimated mean *V. vulnificus* dose per serving was matched with each month- and year-specific number of reported cases, and the modelled relationship was between mean risk and mean dose rather than individual-level risk versus individual-level dose (see Appendix C). The numbers of reported month- and year-specific cases of septicaemia used in this dose-response assessment were those occurring and reported to CDC between 1995 and 2001 (M. Glatzer, personal communication, 2002). Reported cases prior to 1995 were not used since the extent of under-reporting may have been more substantial prior to 1995.

Based upon the estimated doses and epidemiological data, Beta-Poisson and Exponential curve fits were obtained by maximum likelihood. Since the number of servings consumed is large relative to the number of illnesses reported in any given month and year, a Poisson regression approach was used as an appropriate approximation to a Binomial regression. The Exponential model, although not statistically rejected, did not otherwise provide a satisfactory fit to the data and was therefore not considered further with respect to risk characterization (see Appendix C).

An uncertainty analysis of the Beta-Poisson fit was obtained by generating 100 alternative data sets representing uncertainty or variability in the number of cases that could potentially occur in a given month and year and the uncertainty of estimated month- and year-specific mean *V. vulnificus* numbers at harvest. The exposure assessment utilized a quadratic regression to predict *V. vulnificus* numbers versus temperature. The asymptotic standard errors and correlations between the parameter estimates in this regression model were used to define a multinormal uncertainty distribution for the parameters determining mean $\log_{10}$ *V. vulnificus* numbers versus water temperature, and the residual variation of $\log_{10}$ *V. vulnificus* numbers independent of temperature.

Monte Carlo samples from this distribution were used to generate alternative sets of month- and year-specific mean ingested dose by applying the same harvest-to-consumption calculations discussed above. The effect of uncertainty in growth and survival rates post-harvest was not considered. In consideration of potential uncertainties in case reporting and the variability in number of cases that could occur under identical exposure conditions, the uncertainty of month- and year-specific risk estimates was characterized by varying month-

**Table 13**. Estimated monthly mean *V. vulnificus* per gram and *V. vulnificus* per serving at time of consumption based on environmental (water temperature) data versus average USA case burden based on epidemiological reporting data for *V. vulnificus*.

| Month | Mean and std deviation of water temperature (°C)[1] | Mean $log_{10}$ *V. vulnificus*/g | | Landings (kg)[2] | Total meals | Servings for at-risk individuals | *V. vulnificus*/serving (dose) | | Average no. of Cases[3] |
|---|---|---|---|---|---|---|---|---|---|
| | | At harvest | At consumption | | | | Median | Mean | |
| Jan | 12.9 (2.9) | 0.06 | -0.11 | 719 398 | 1 835 000 | 128 000 | 155 | 14 000 | 0.14 |
| Feb | 15.1 (2.8) | 0.73 | 0.65 | 737 541 | 1 882 000 | 132 000 | 890 | 70 000 | 0.14 |
| Mar | 17.4 (2.0) | 1.41 | 1.47 | 847 311 | 2 162 000 | 151 000 | 6 000 | 109 000 | 0.29 |
| Apr | 21.7 (1.7) | 2.36 | 2.68 | 733 459 | 1 871 000 | 131 000 | 94 900 | 675 000 | 1.86 |
| May | 25.8 (1.9) | 2.98 | 3.65 | 616 432 | 1 573 000 | 110 000 | 888 000 | 5 025 000 | 4.57 |
| Jun | 28.8 (1.4) | 3.26 | 4.15 | 588 309 | 1 501 000 | 105 000 | 2 855 000 | 11 561 000 | 3.14 |
| Jul | 30.0 (1.2) | 3.32 | 4.31 | 542 043 | 1 383 000 | 97 000 | 4 095 000 | 15 598 000 | 4.14 |
| Aug | 30.3 (1.0) | 3.33 | 4.33 | 492 148 | 1 256 000 | 88 000 | 4 231 000 | 16 536 000 | 5.14 |
| Sep | 28.2 (1.7) | 3.21 | 4.02 | 555 197 | 1 416 000 | 99 000 | 2 074 000 | 9 008 000 | 4.71 |
| Oct | 22.7 (2.7) | 2.51 | 2.94 | 710 779 | 1 813 000 | 127 000 | 173 000 | 1 943 000 | 4.43 |
| Nov | 18.4 (2.8) | 1.64 | 1.71 | 817 827 | 2 086 000 | 146 000 | 10 300 | 257 000 | 2.71 |
| Dec | 15.4 (2.5) | 0.84 | 0.77 | 835 064 | 2 130 000 | 149 000 | 1 170 | 39 000 | 0.71 |

NOTES: (1) Average monthly water temperatures at Dauphin Island and Weeks Bay, Alabama, USA, 1995–2001. (2) Average 1990–1998. (3) Based on confirmed illnesses 1995–2000.

and year-specific case incidence as a Poisson random variable with mean equal to the month- and year-specific case incidence reported to the CDC.

Figures 10 and 11 show the maximum likelihood estimate of the Beta-Poisson dose-response curve for *V. vulnificus* septicaemia. The dots represent the best estimates of the month- and year-specific exposure based on water temperatures and the risk of illness based on the observed epidemiology (1995–2001). The solid line is the most likely Beta-Poisson model and the parallel dashed lines are 90% upper and lower uncertainty limits on the predicted risk based on the uncertainty factors identified and considered here. Figure 10, which illustrates the relationship between log risk and log dose, excludes instances for which the reported number of month- and year-specific cases was zero. However, estimated data points with zero reported cases still influence the maximum likelihood fit of the Beta-Poisson curve, as indicated by the fact that the curve and confidence interval are substantially below the data points plotted for exposures less that $10^5$.

Figure 11 showing the relationship between risk and $\log_{10}$ dose indicates the influence of the estimated data points for which the reported number of cases was zero. The best estimates of the parameters for the Beta-Poisson model are $\alpha = 9.3 \times 10^{-6}$ and $\beta = 110\,000$. A Monte Carlo uncertainty sample of the alpha and beta parameters of the Beta-Poisson model resulting from the identified uncertainties of exposure and risk is shown in Figure 12. As is evident from this sample, the confidence region for $\log(\alpha)$ and $\log(\beta)$ is an ellipsoid with strong correlation between uncertainty of $\log(\alpha)$ and $\log(\beta)$.

### 4.3.3. Assumptions

In developing the dose-response model for *V. vulnificus*, the following assumptions were made:

- the mean meal size is 196 g per serving;
- seven percent of the population is at risk (Klontz, 1997) and this population consumes raw oysters with the same frequency as non-susceptible individuals;
- the estimated mean number of *V. vulnificus* cells per gram at consumption is based on a regression equation for $\log_{10}$ *V. vulnificus*/g versus temperature at harvest, average time unrefrigerated, estimated growth rate versus temperature, and survival in cold storage;
- the estimates of monthly mean *V. vulnificus* per serving, based on the exposure analysis conducted, are assumed accurate. These estimates are based on the assumption that no temperature abuse occurs after oysters reach no-growth temperatures; and
- the use of mean *V. vulnificus*/g rather than median *V. vulnificus*/g (i.e. mean $\log_{10}$ *V. vulnificus*/g) as a summary measure of exposure for a group is considered appropriate for dose-response analysis (i.e. for grouped data with varying individual doses within each group it is considered more appropriate to relate the average response to average (mean) dose).

### 4.3.4. Goodness of fit

The goodness of fit of the dose-response models considered (Beta-Poisson and Exponential) was assessed based on the Deviance (McCullagh and Nelder, 1989), which is a likelihood ratio statistic contrasting the maximum likelihood attained under a specified model compared with the maximum possible likelihood, without any constraint. Although both dose-response models were found to provide adequate fit statistically, the fit of the Exponential model was found to be appreciably worse than that of the Beta-Poisson (see Appendix C).

### 4.3.5. Uncertainty and variability

This analysis incorporates both uncertainty and variability in the estimates.

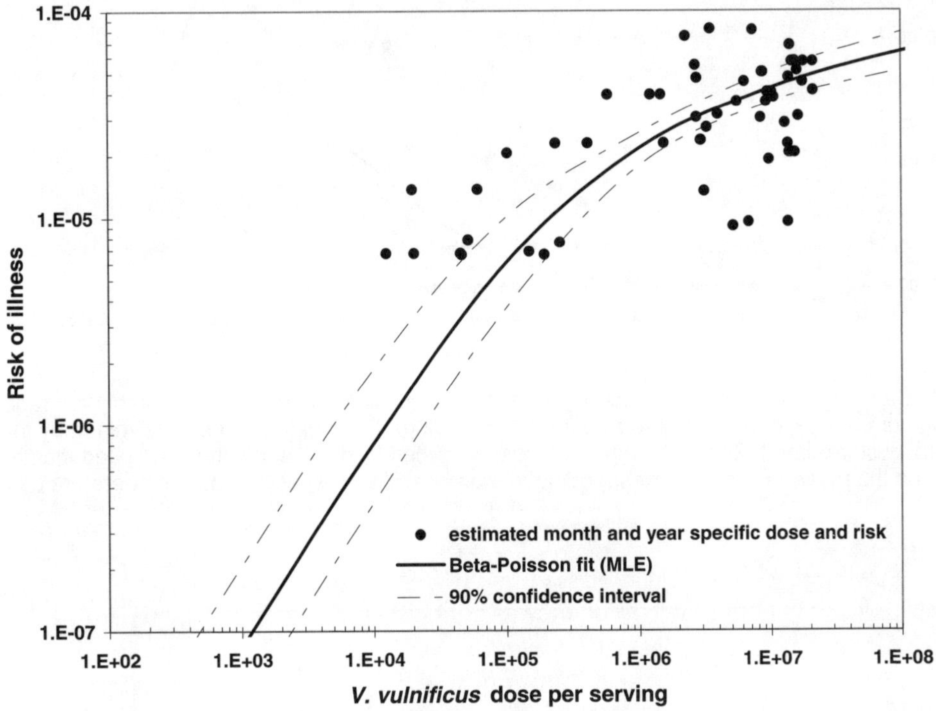


**Figure 10**. Log-log plot of Beta-Poisson dose-response curve for *V. vulnificus* ($\log_{10}$ of monthly average risk per serving versus $\log_{10}$ of monthly average dose per serving). Each point is determined by the risk of reported oyster-related illness (number of observed cases divided by the estimated number of servings) and the mean exposure corresponding to month- and year-specific water temperature data.

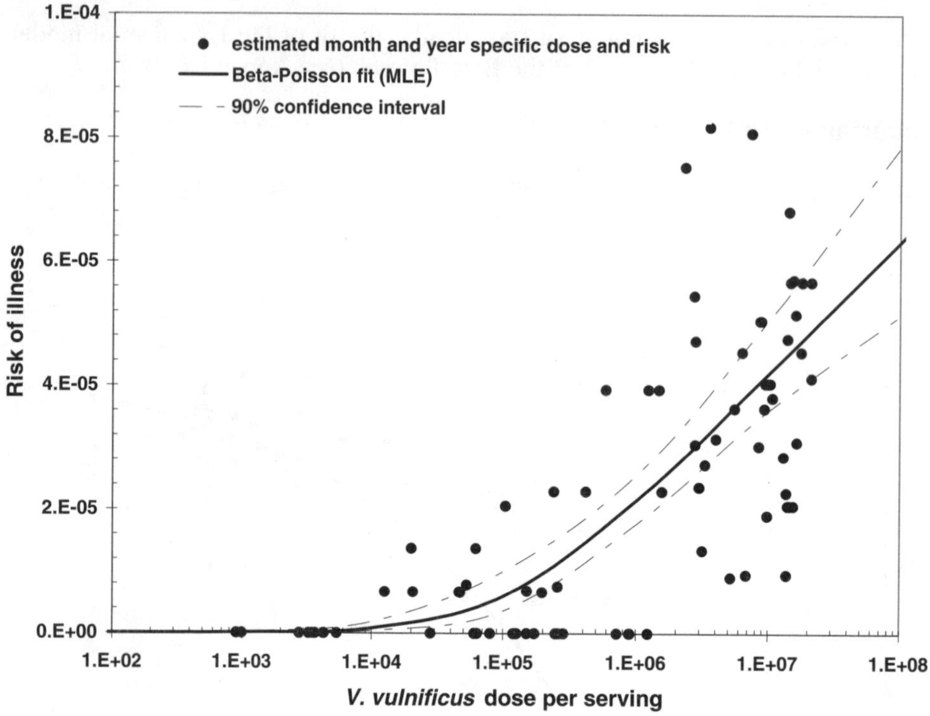


**Figure 11**. Semi-log plot of Beta-Poisson dose-response curve for *V. vulnificus* (monthly average risk per serving versus $\log_{10}$ of monthly average dose per serving). Each data point is determined by the risk of reported oyster-related illness (number of observed cases divided by the estimated number of servings) and the mean exposure corresponding to month- and year-specific water temperature data.

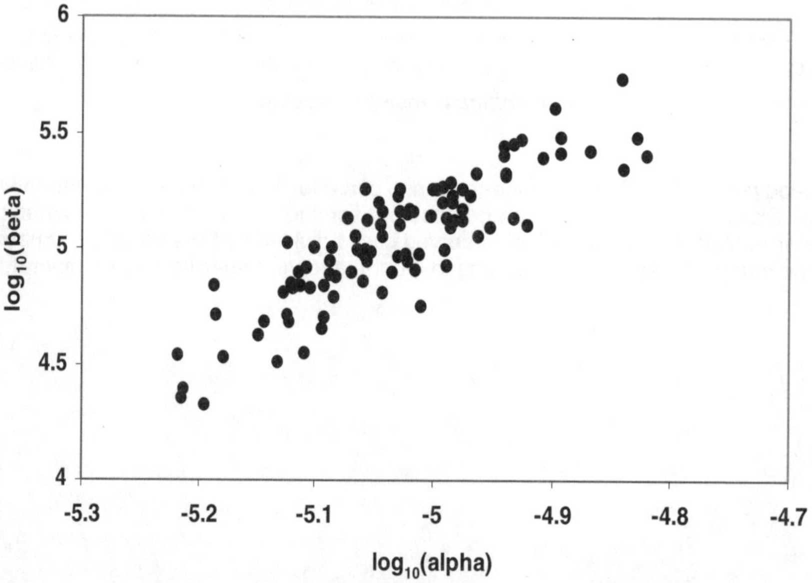


**Figure 12**. Parameter uncertainty of the Beta-Poisson dose-response model fit to *V. vulnificus* epidemiological data and estimated month- and year-specific mean exposure.

# 5. Risk characterization

## 5.1. Moderate salinity

Baseline risk characterization results for *V. vulnificus* in raw oysters are shown in Table 14. This characterization of exposure and risk was based on use of the Motes et al. (averaged) data for assessment of *V. vulnificus* densities versus water temperature at the time of harvest. Additional analyses based on alternative data sources were evaluated and are discussed in Appendix D. The model-based predictions of *V. vulnificus* densities in oysters at the time of consumption and the number of illnesses for each season of the year were based on current industry practices and estimates of the typical (average) daily mean and variance of water temperatures within the different seasons. These temperatures were determined from aggregate coastal water temperature measurements collected from 1995 to 2001 at Dauphin Bay, Alabama, on the USA Gulf Coast, and were assumed to be representative of the Gulf Coast region as a whole. Gaps in the dataset as a result of Hurricane Georges in 1998 were completed with data from other bays in the region. Table 14 presents the predicted mean $\log_{10}$ *V. vulnificus*/g and the mean *V. vulnificus*/g with respect to both time of harvest and time of consumption. The seasonal differences in the change of *V. vulnificus*/g at consumption versus harvest are a consequence of the relative effects of time unrefrigerated and ambient air temperature. Additional risk characterizations were conducted that were specific to the autumn of 1998 and the winter of 1999. These results are also shown in Table 14. These specific periods were selected to examine the effect of the higher than normal air and water temperatures that existed in the USA Gulf Coast region at that time. This approach is consistent with increasing recognition being given to the effect of atypical climatic events on the incidence of infectious disease (Rose, Huq and Lipp, 1999). The higher temperatures were a consequence of a strong La Nina event that occurred over continental USA from the autumn of 1998 to the spring of 1999. Additionally, a market study of *V. parahaemolyticus* and *V. vulnificus* levels in oysters from USA retail establishments was conducted in the period from June 1998 to June 1999 (Cook et al., 2002). Thus, empirical data exists that is specific to *V. vulnificus* levels in market oysters during the period of the La Nina and provides a basis for assessing the accuracy of model-based predictions.

With respect to the baseline assessment, using typical seasonal water temperature parameters (Motes et al., 1998), the predicted mean numbers of illnesses were 0.5, 11.7, 12.2 and 8.0 for the winter (January – March), spring (April – June), summer (July – September) and autumn (October – December) seasons, respectively. These predictions were based on the seasonal estimates of mean risk per serving and the estimated number of servings consumed, as shown in Table 13. Uncertainty ranges associated with these estimates were determined based on the identified uncertainties in *V. vulnificus*/g at harvest versus water temperature and the dose-response. The central 90% uncertainty ranges are shown in Table 14 for risk per serving and the expected number of illness, as well as *V. vulnificus*/g at harvest and at time of consumption. With respect to the number of illnesses, the 90% uncertainty range for the total annual number of illnesses is a >2-fold range from 25.9 to 42.8, with a mean of 32.4.

**Table 14.** Summary output of the seasonal predictions based on the risk assessment simulation: mean and 90% uncertainty intervals for exposure (*V. vulnificus*/g at harvest and at time of consumption) and risk (risk per serving and number of cases given the estimated number of servings consumed, based on data in Table 13).

| Month | $Log_{10}$ *V. vulnificus*/g at harvest | *V. vulnificus*/g at harvest | $Log_{10}$ *V. vulnificus*/g at consumption | *V. vulnificus*/g at consumption | Risk per serving for at-risk population | Predicted no. of cases[2] |
|---|---|---|---|---|---|---|
| Winter | 0.47 | 40 | 0.30 | 80 | $1.26\times10^{-6}$ | 0.5 |
| (Jan. – Mar.) | (-0.39, 1.04) | (10, 140) | (-0.60, 1.01) | (20, 610) | ($2.92\times10^{-7}$, $6.71\times10^{-6}$) | (0.1, 2.8) |
| Spring | 2.75 | 2 600 | 3.28 | 21 400 | $3.37\times10^{-5}$ | 11.7 |
| (Apr. – Jun.) | (2.39, 2.97) | (1 600, 3 900) | (2.80, 3.61) | (12 700, 33 500) | ($2.83\times10^{-5}$, $4.05\times10^{-5}$) | (9.8, 14.0) |
| Summer | 3.27 | 5 600 | 4.15 | 57 000 | $4.28\times10^{-5}$ | 12.2 |
| (Jul. – Sep.) | (3.09, 3.41) | (3 200, 7 800) | (3.95, 4.29) | (37 900, 70 500) | ($3.69\times10^{-5}$, $4.97\times10^{-5}$) | (10.5, 14.1) |
| Autumn | 1.39 | 500 | 1.45 | 3 700 | $1.92\times10^{-5}$ | 8.0 |
| (Oct. – Dec.) | (0.33, 2.06) | (220, 1 100) | (0.26, 2.32) | (1 500, 11 700) | ($1.30\times10^{-5}$, $2.82\times10^{-5}$) | (5.5, 11.9) |
| Autumn 1998 [1] | 2.54 | 1 700 | 2.99 | 16 100 | $3.11\times10^{-5}$ | 13.1 |
| | (2.41, 2.68) | (1 100, 2 400) | (2.86, 3.12) | (11 800, 19 800) | ($2.78\times10^{-5}$, $3.57\times10^{-5}$) | (11.7, 15.0) |
| Winter 1999 [1] | 1.11 | 110 | 1.08 | 390 | $4.87\times10^{-6}$ | 2.0 |
| | (0.90, 1.31) | (80, 170) | (0.87, 1.28) | (240, 590) | ($2.93\times10^{-6}$, $7.74\times10^{-6}$) | (1.2, 3.2) |

NOTES: (1) Predictions based on water temperature distributions for Weeks Bay, Alabama, USA, in 1998 and 1999.
(2) Based on number of servings (data from Table 13).

For six of the seven years (1995–2001) the number of reported cases was within the 90% confidence limit predicted by the model; in 1997 there were 21 reported cases. These predictions are based on a dose-response derived from the total cases of *V. vulnificus* illness (224 cases) identified between 1995 and 2001 within the continental USA (M. Glatzer, personal communication, 2001) and thus the predictions are generally in good agreement with the values in Table 13. Most, though not all, of these cases were definitively associated with the consumption of oysters harvested from the USA Gulf Coast. This suggests an average annual illness rate of 32 cases.

Predicted *V. vulnificus* levels and cases are compared with *V. vulnificus* levels reported in the market study and reported cases for each month of the year (Table C.4 in Appendix C). The *V. vulnificus* levels in market oysters were considerably higher in the autumn of 1998 than predicted by the baseline risk characterization, which was based on normal water temperatures. The water and air temperatures used for the risk characterization were derived from aggregate data recorded at the NBDC buoy located at Dauphin Island, Alabama, on the USA Gulf Coast, with missing data filled in from the nearby NERRS site (Weeks Bay) from the years 1995 to 2001 (Table 15). The temperatures observed in the autumn of 1998 were approximately 4°C higher than the mean temperature used in the risk assessment (Tables 15 and 16). Repeating the simulations for this period using the 1998-specific buoy observations results in much closer agreement with the *V. vulnificus* levels observed in the market study (See Figure 9 in Section 3). The predicted seasonal illnesses in Table 14 agree well with the observed or reported illnesses, as presented in Table 17, considering either the average number of illnesses between 1995 and 2001 or in the autumn of 1998 and winter of 1999.

**Table 15.** Mean and range of average water temperatures (°C) at selected sites on the USA Gulf Coast (1995–2001 data).

| Season | Average water temperature (°C) – mean and range | |
|---|---|---|
| | Recorded at NBDC buoy located at Dauphin Island, Alabama | Recorded at NERRS site at Weeks Bay, Alabama |
| Winter | 15.0 (14.0 – 16.2) | 15.4 (13.6 – 17.4) |
| Spring | 25.1 (23.8 – 26.1) | 25.8 (24.5 – 26.5) |
| Summer | 29.6 (29.4 – 29.7) | 29.7 (29.5 – 30.0) |
| Autumn | 19.4 (17.6 – 22.3) | 19.0 (17.2 – 23.0) |

NOTE: (1) There is missing data from both stations in 1995 and data is missing from Dauphin Island from winter of 1999 through the end of 2001.

**Table 16** Average water temperatures (°C) at selected sites on the USA Gulf Coast during the time of the ISSC/FDA market survey of *V. parahaemolyticus* and *V. vulnificus* levels at point of sale.

| Season and Year | Average water temperature (°C) | |
|---|---|---|
| | Recorded at NBDC buoy located at Dauphin Island, Alabama | Recorded at NERRS site at Weeks Bay, Alabama |
| Spring 1998 | 25.5 | 26.5 |
| Summer 1998 | 29.7 | 30.0 |
| Autumn 1998 | 22.3 | 23.0 |
| Winter 1999 | n.a. | 16.4 |
| Spring 1999 | n.a. | 25.9 |
| Summer 1999 | n.a. | 29.5 |

NOTE: n.a. = No data available at Dauphin Island from winter 1999 to summer 1999.

**Table 17.** Average seasonal illness rates in 1995–2001 compared with 1998 and 1999 (There was a La Nina event from autumn 1998 to spring 1999).

| Season | Average no. of illnesses observed (1995-2001) | No. of illnesses observed in 1998 | No. of illnesses observed in 1999 |
|---|---|---|---|
| Winter | 0.6 | 0 | 2 |
| Spring | 9.6 | 13 | 10 |
| Summer | 13.5 | 10 | 18 |
| Autumn | 7.4 | 17 | 4 |

## 5.2. Effects of interventions

The predicted reduction of illness that could be achieved by post-harvest treatments or other means to reduce *V. vulnificus* levels to various targeted values is presented in Table 18. There are currently three approaches that have been validated for post-harvest processing of oysters in the USA to achieve an end-point criterion of < 3 MPN/g and using such a process allows the product to be labelled as "Processed to reduce *Vibrio vulnificus* to non-detectable levels" (DHHS, 1999). These processes include mild heat (50°C) treatment; freezing, with extended frozen storage; and high hydrostatic pressure. Using the Motes et al. (averaged) data as a basis for prediction, such a process would reduce the number of cases from a current level of around 32 reported cases in the USA per year to approximately one case every six years if all oysters intended for raw consumption were treated. If the targeted goal were shifted to 30 or 300 MPN/g, then the number of cases would increase to 1.2 and 7.7 cases per year, respectively. The predicted reductions vary considerably depending on the data selected for exposure assessment, with the smallest reductions being predicted based on the Motes et al. (averaged) data and the largest based on the Tamplin data (see Appendix D). However, the model predictions based on the Motes et al. (averaged) data are in closest agreement with the retail data (Table 11), especially during the winter, when levels are closest to the targeted mitigation levels.

Table 19 illustrates the effect of time unrefrigerated on expected numbers of illnesses. Predicted annual illnesses ranged from 17.7 to 59.3 for time unrefrigerated ranging from 0 to 20 hours. Thus, immediate cooling of all oysters intended for raw consumption alone may not be sufficient to achieve a substantial reduction in *V. vulnificus* illnesses. However, further reduction in illnesses would probably occur if the temperature were reduced rapidly (i.e. icing on board), as the predictions in Table 19 assume a 1- to 10-hour cool-down time to reach 13°C (no-growth temperature for *V. vulnificus*).

In 1996, the National Shellfish Sanitation Program (NSSP) time-temperature matrix for control of *V. vulnificus* went into effect in the USA. Oyster harvesters from any state that previously had two or more confirmed cases of *V. vulnificus* were required to place oysters under refrigeration within 10 hours after harvest during summer months, depending on water temperature (DHHS, 1999). A dealer survey of industry practices prior to and immediately following the adoption of this requirement (Cook, 1997b) indicates that the actual times to refrigeration changed minimally as a result of this control measure: from a maximum of 12 hours to 9 hours in Louisiana, and from a maximum of 9 hours to 8 hours in other states on the Gulf Coast of the USA (Table 20). In addition to the maximum time, the dealer survey also included self-reported statistics as to the minimum and most likely duration of harvesting, from which an estimate of the distributions was inferred by fitting the Beta-PERT distribution. Based on the resulting estimates of the distribution of time unrefrigerated prior to and after 1996, the current model indicates that the mean time to refrigeration was only reduced from 5.27 to 5.13 hours and that only 1–2 cases/year have been prevented (Table 21). This confirmed the earlier observations (Table 19) that small reductions in the period of time to refrigeration after harvest had a limited effect in terms of reducing illnesses.

**Table 18.** Predicted mean and 90% uncertainty intervals for risk per serving and annual number of illnesses for three alternative process target levels.

| Data used to estimate the *V. vulnificus*/g versus water temperature relationship (at harvest) | Target | Mean risk per serving (median and 90% interval of uncertainty distribution) | Predicted annual number of cases (median and 90% interval of uncertainty distribution)(1) |
|---|---|---|---|
| Motes et al., 1998 (averaged) | 3/g | $1.09 \times 10^{-7}$ ($4.10 \times 10^{-8}$, $2.73 \times 10^{-7}$) | 0.16 (0.06, 0.4) |
| Motes et al., 1998 (averaged) | 30/g | $8.20 \times 10^{-7}$ ($3.42 \times 10^{-7}$, $2.12 \times 10^{-6}$) | 1.2 (0.5, 3.1) |
| Motes et al., 1998 (averaged) | 300/g | $5.26 \times 10^{-6}$ ($2.60 \times 10^{-6}$, $1.05 \times 10^{-6}$) | 7.7 (3.8, 15.3) |

NOTE: (1) Based on an estimated annual consumption rate of 1 464 000 servings by immunocompromised individuals (data from Table 13).

**Table 19.** Effect of time unrefrigerated on $\log_{10}$ *V. vulnificus* levels, risk per serving and expected number of illnesses (mean predictions and 90% uncertainty intervals based on uncertainty of the $\log_{10}$ *V. vulnificus*/g versus water temperature relationship at harvest and year-to-year water temperature variations).

| Season | Time to first refrigeration(3) | Mean $\log_{10}$ *V. vulnificus*/g at consumption | Mean risk per serving(1) | Expected no. of cases(2) |
|---|---|---|---|---|
| Winter | 0 hr | 0.21 (-0.66, 0.83) | $4.7 \times 10^{-7}$ ($1.4 \times 10^{-7}$, $1.7 \times 10^{-6}$) | 0.19 (0.06, 0.68) |
| | 5 hr | 0.30 (-0.60, 1.01) | $9.7 \times 10^{-7}$ ($2.3 \times 10^{-7}$, $4.8 \times 10^{-6}$) | 0.40 (0.09, 1.96) |
| | 10 hr | 0.38 (-0.54, 1.14) | $2.6 \times 10^{-6}$ ($5.5 \times 10^{-7}$, $1.1 \times 10^{-5}$) | 1.08 (0.23, 4.45) |
| | 20 hr | 0.57 (-0.42, 1.44) | $7.3 \times 10^{-6}$ ($3.9 \times 10^{-6}$, $1.3 \times 10^{-5}$) | 5.12 (1.29, 11.05) |
| Spring | 0 hr | 2.79 (2.40, 3.06) | $2.0 \times 10^{-5}$ ($1.5 \times 10^{-5}$, $2.4 \times 10^{-5}$) | 6.77 (5.27, 8.45) |
| | 5 hr | 3.35 (2.86, 3.68) | $3.4 \times 10^{-5}$ ($2.8 \times 10^{-5}$, $4.1 \times 10^{-5}$) | 11.59 (9.78, 14.08) |
| | 10 hr | 3.89 (3.29, 4.27) | $4.5 \times 10^{-5}$ ($3.9 \times 10^{-5}$, $5.4 \times 10^{-5}$) | 15.48 (13.49, 18.82) |
| | 20 hr | 4.69 (3.97, 5.10) | $1.8 \times 10^{-5}$ ($1.1 \times 10^{-5}$, $2.5 \times 10^{-5}$) | 19.28 (16.11, 24.06) |
| Summer | 0 hr | 3.46 (3.28, 3.60) | $2.7 \times 10^{-5}$ ($2.3 \times 10^{-5}$, $3.1 \times 10^{-5}$) | 7.65 (6.57, 8,82) |
| | 5 hr | 4.24 (4.04, 4.38) | $4.3 \times 10^{-5}$ ($3.7 \times 10^{-5}$, $4.9 \times 10^{-5}$) | 12.16 (10.46, 14.04) |
| | 10 hr | 4.94 (4.75, 5.07) | $5.4 \times 10^{-5}$ ($4.6 \times 10^{-5}$, $6.5 \times 10^{-5}$) | 15.31 (12.93, 18.34) |
| | 20 hr | 5.61 (5.55, 5.65) | $2.8 \times 10^{-5}$ ($2.1 \times 10^{-5}$, $3.7 \times 10^{-5}$) | 17.55 (15.51, 21.66) |
| Autumn | 0 hr | 1.23 (0.12, 1.97) | $7.3 \times 10^{-6}$ ($3.9 \times 10^{-6}$, $1.3 \times 10^{-5}$) | 3.06 (1.64, 5.46) |
| | 5 hr | 1.45 (0.26, 2.32) | $1.8 \times 10^{-5}$ ($1.1 \times 10^{-6}$, $2.5 \times 10^{-5}$) | 7.37 (4.66, 10.62) |
| | 10 hr | 1.68 (0.41, 2.65) | $2.8 \times 10^{-5}$ ($2.1 \times 10^{-5}$, $3.7 \times 10^{-5}$) | 11.64 (8.91, 15.72) |
| | 20 hr | 2.09 (0.69, 3.22) | $4.1 \times 10^{-5}$ ($3.3 \times 10^{-5}$, $5.2 \times 10^{-5}$) | 17.30 (13.72, 21.98) |

NOTES: (1) Based on 1 000 Monte Carlo samples for each of 100 uncertainty samples for the $\log_{10}$ *V. vulnificus* versus water temperature relationship and year-to-year water temperature differences.
(2) Expected cases based on 411 000, 346 000, 284 000 and 422 000 servings for the winter, spring, summer and autumn seasons, respectively.
(3) Duration from harvest until oysters are first placed under refrigeration; normal cooling with a range of 1 to 10 hours until no-growth temperature (13°C) is reached was assumed.

**Table 20**. Duration of harvesting estimates used in the risk assessment.

| Season | Louisiana pre-1996 change | Louisiana post-1996 change | Other states pre-1996 change | Other states post-1996 change |
|---|---|---|---|---|
| Spring and summer | Min = 7<br>Max = 13<br>Mode = 12 | Min = 5<br>Max = 11<br>Mode = 9 | Min = 2<br>Max = 11<br>Mode = 8 | Min = 3<br>Max = 10<br>Mode = 7 |
| Winter and autumn | Min = 7<br>Max = 13<br>Mode = 12 | Min = 7<br>Max = 13<br>Mode = 12 | Min = 2<br>Max = 11<br>Mode = 8 | Min = 2<br>Max = 11<br>Mode = 8 |

NOTE: Minimum, maximum and mode (most likely) estimates of the duration of harvesting (in hours) were used to define Beta-PERT distributions used in model simulations; only the spring and summer harvests were determined to be associated with high enough water temperatures (in a typical year) for the new guidelines to become standard practice; winter and autumn harvests were assumed unaffected.

**Table 21.** Predicted effects of 1996 reductions in time unrefrigerated requirement.

| Season | Time unrefrigerated | Mean and std deviation of time unrefrigerated | Mean and std deviation of $\log_{10}$ *V. vulnificus*/g at consumption | Expected no. of cases(1) |
|---|---|---|---|---|
| Spring | Pre1996 change | 5.27 (2.81) | 3.36 (1.11) | 12.6 (10.7, 15.2) |
| Spring | Post-1996 change | 5.13 (2.77) | 3.27 (1.08) | 11.7 (9.8, 14.0) |
| Summer | Pre-1996 change | 5.27 (2.81) | 4.25 (0.81) | 12.9 (11.1, 15.0) |
| Summer | Post-1996 change | 5.13 (2.77) | 4.12 (0.78) | 12.2 (10.5, 14.1) |

NOTE: (1) Median and 90% interval of uncertainty distribution.

## 5.3. High salinity

As discussed in the exposure assessment section, *V. vulnificus* levels in oysters at harvest are substantially reduced at high (>30 ppt) compared with moderate (<30 ppt) salinities. Conservative estimates of the mean at-harvest *V. vulnificus* levels were obtained based on the high salinity data by taking simple arithmetic averages after replacing non-detectable outcomes by half the limit of detection. In order to estimate at-consumption densities and a corresponding estimate of risk, post-harvest growth estimates are also needed. However, there is little information available about growth rates of *V. vulnificus* in oysters harvested from high salinity waters and the assumption of growth similar to that in oysters harvested at moderate salinity may not be valid. Growth in oysters harvested from high salinity areas would be expected to be minimal since these conditions result in remarkably lower levels of the pathogen than those observed at moderate salinities.

Given this identified uncertainty with respect to growth at high salinities and already conservative estimates of *V. vulnificus* levels at harvest, best estimates of *V. vulnificus* densities at consumption in oysters harvested from high salinity waters were not developed. Instead, an uncertainty range of at-consumption densities was obtained by considering the extremes of growth that might occur. This uncertainty range was defined by assuming that either growth post-harvest is zero or equal to that occurring in oysters harvested from moderate salinity waters.

The resulting uncertainty range for *V. vulnificus* levels at consumption is given in Table 22 based on initial at-harvest levels as determined based on the Motes et al. high-salinity data. A similar analysis of the Tokyo Bay data would require data on post-harvest practices in Japan, since post-harvest handling practices specific to the USA might not be applicable. The lower limit of the uncertainty range of densities at consumption presented in Table 22 assumes that there is no growth from harvest to consumption and an average of 0.31 logs of die-off during storage (i.e. the die-off rate times the mean duration of storage of 7.7 days). This corresponds to a 5-fold reduction in mean *V. vulnificus*/g. The upper limit of the range assumes that the relative difference in *V. vulnificus*/g at consumption versus at harvest is the same for high salinity as for moderate salinity. The results of the seasonal simulations (Table 9) were used to obtain these relative differences. Based on the simulations, the relative increase of consumption levels compared with at-harvest levels averages 2-fold, 8.2-fold, 10.2-fold, and 7.4-fold for the winter, spring, summer and autumn, respectively. Based on the mean seasonal water temperatures in comparison with the temperature ranges in Table 22, a 7.4-fold higher difference was taken to correspond to the <20°C range and 10.2-fold difference was assumed for all temperature ranges >20°C. An uncertainty range for mean risk per serving was then obtained by multiplying the uncertainty range of at-consumption densities by a mean serving size of 196 g and using the MLE of the Beta-Poisson dose-response to obtain a corresponding risk.

The results of the calculations, as presented in Table 22, indicate that the risk of *V. vulnificus* infection from consumption of raw oysters harvested from growing areas with salinities >30 ppt is greatly reduced (<1 illness per year at all the temperature ranges, assuming all raw oyster consumption was from growing waters with >30 ppt salinity) in comparison with oysters harvested from moderate-salinity growing areas, regardless of temperature. It should be noted that the growth of *V. vulnificus* in high-salinity oysters has not been reported and hence the lower limit of the uncertainty range for risk may be regarded as more likely than the upper limit of the uncertainty range.

**Table 22.** Risk estimates for United States oysters harvested from high salinity (>30 ppt) areas (USA Atlantic and Gulf Coast data, Motes et al., 1998).

| Salinity range | Temperature range | Mean *V. vulnificus*/g at harvest | Uncertainty range for mean *V. vulnificus*/g at consumption | Uncertainty range for corresponding risk per serving(1) |
|---|---|---|---|---|
| >30 ppt | < 20°C | 2.8 | (0.6, 21) | ($1.0 \times 10^{-8}$, $3.4 \times 10^{-7}$) |
| >30 ppt | 20–25°C | 19.5 | (3.9, 200) | ($6.5 \times 10^{-8}$, $2.9 \times 10^{-6}$) |
| >30 ppt | 25–30°C | 2.7 | (0.5, 28) | ($8.3 \times 10^{-9}$, $4.6 \times 10^{-7}$) |
| >30 ppt | >30°C | 4.2 | (0.8, 43) | ($1.3 \times 10^{-8}$, $6.9 \times 10^{-7}$) |

Note: (1) Based on MLE of the dose-response ($\log(\alpha) = -5.03$, $\log(\beta) = 5.04$) and a mean of 196 g per serving

# 6. Data gaps

In the USA, especially for the Gulf Coast region, there are data available for each of the model inputs. However, outside of that country there is a scarcity of useful data for quantitative risk assessment of *V. vulnificus,* including information on the numbers of *V. vulnificus* in foods, consumption patterns and epidemiology. Recent reports suggest that *V. vulnificus* may be of equivalent, if not greater, importance in some Asian countries. In the Republic of Korea, for example, a single hospital reported 49 *V. vulnificus* primary septicaemia cases in five years that were generally associated with consumption of raw shellfish and fish (Park, Shon and Joh, 1991). Five hospitals in Taiwan reported 18 *V. vulnificus* primary septicaemia cases over approximately a five-year period, but provided little information on incriminated seafood's (Chuang et al., 1992). Several *V. vulnificus* cases were also reported in Thailand (Thamlikitkul, 1990). A recent survey of Kumamoto Prefecture in Japan detected 6 cases of *V. vulnificus* primary septicaemia during a 20-day period from 29 June–18 July 2001 (Ono, Inoue and Yokoyama, 2001). Seafood products other than molluscan shellfish may also be important vehicles for transmission of *V. vulnificus* septicaemia and three fatal cases in Kumamoto Prefecture, Japan were attributed to consumption of raw flathead fish that had been marinated in soy source for one day (Ono, Inoue and Yokoyama, 2001).

While the risk assessment is relatively complete for one geographic area, a number of questions arose in the course of this work that need to be addressed in order to provide data to reduce the number of assumptions that had to be made and to expand this work to other geographic areas. They questions are as follows:

- Are all *V. vulnificus* strains equally virulent?

This issue has been addressed by two studies (Nilsson et al., 2003; DePaola et al., 2003). One study found that 25 clinical isolates could not be distinguished from 25 market oyster isolates by plasmid profile, RAPD-PCR patterns or in a mouse (subcutaneous injected) virulence model (DePaola et al., 2003). However, a similar study looked at the presence of type A and B 16S rRNA genes using the same *V. vulnificus* culture collection and some additional isolates. Type B 16S rRNA genes were identified in 74% of clinical isolates and only 6% of the oyster isolates (Nilsson et al., 2003). While the current risk assessment made the assumption that all strains are equally virulent these latter findings could affect the outcome of the risk characterization if the distribution of types A and B *V. vulnificus* varied by season. More data will be needed before this could be addressed in the risk assessment but already one survey on *V. vulnificus* in oysters in the Republic of Korea indicated that the frequency of type B was 65% (Kim and Jeong, 2001).

- If *V. vulnificus* strains vary in virulence, how can degrees of virulence be assigned to various subpopulations within the population in oysters?

It may be possible to assign degrees of virulence based on a ratio of frequency of type A or B 16S rRNA genes in clinical cases versus oysters that could be used as multiplier (i.e. if type B occurs at a frequency of 0.74 in clinical isolates and 0.06 in market oysters, then the ratio would be 0.74/0.06 = 12.33, whereas the corresponding ratio of type A would be 0.26/0.94 = 0.28). These data suggest that the type B is 44 (12.33/0.28) times more virulent than type A. Thus, samples or months that had a higher frequency of the type B could be weighted to have greater risk.

- Does virulence vary by season, region or source (shellfish, finfish, water, etc.)?

The prevalence of type B 16S rRNA genes was 10-fold higher in *V. vulnificus* isolates from Republic of Korea oysters (65%) compared with those from the USA (6%), but only 40 and 33 oyster isolates were examined, respectively, in these studies (Nilsson et al., 2003; Kim and Jeong, 2001). Thus more data will be needed in order to be more conclusive on this question.

- Are all members of the at-risk population equally susceptible?

As data relevant to addressing this issue is very limited and it could not really be addressed in the current assessment. The current dose-response approach therefore limits the relevance of this assumption to: Are there seasonal differences in susceptibility of the at-risk population? The monthly incidence of *V. vulnificus* cases used to develop the dose-response relationship was obtained from essentially the same population of at-risk individuals.

- If susceptibility varies among individuals or susceptibility is not constant within an individual, how can the at-risk population be defined and properly weighted for the degree of susceptibility?

This is an issue in particular for countries that may have a significantly different distribution of risk factors among its at-risk population than those considered in this risk assessment. For instance, liver disease is probably a more important factor than diabetes in Southeast Asian countries.

- Is it appropriate to weight susceptibility by a factor of increased incidence of *V. vulnificus* infections in a particular at-risk population?

*V. vulnificus* infections were 4.5 times higher in diabetics than among non-diabetics in a study in Florida in the USA, and it may be possible to determine ratios for other risk factors, such as liver disease, and to use these to weight the risk among various at-risk populations.

- Is there month-to-month bias in reporting of *V. vulnificus* infections within a defined epidemiological region?

Month-to-month bias in reporting would be minimized by having a consistent surveillance system.

- Is the risk of *V. vulnificus* infection dependent on exposure and independent of vehicle of infection?

It is possible that some food matrices might be more or less protective of *V. vulnificus* compared with oysters in relation to factors such as the effect of stomach acidity.

- What are the weaknesses of developing a dose-response relationship based on monthly differences in exposure and reported illnesses within a defined epidemiological unit?

Existence of unidentified seasonal differences in raw consumption patterns or prevalence of more virulent strains could bias results if there were substantial deviation from the assumption of no seasonal differences. Additionally, a dose-response relationship based on aggregate-level data may be biased with respect to individual-level dose versus risk predictions.

- What are the obstacles to applying this dose-response relationship to other foods, regions or countries?

The prevalence of more virulent strains may vary by food or region (as shown by different frequencies of type B rRNA genes in environmental *V. vulnificus* isolates from the USA and Republic of Korea). Different seafood's may vary in protecting *V. vulnificus* from host defences in humans. The proportion of the population at risk and the distribution of risk factors may vary by country or region (i.e. higher frequencies of hepatitis C in Asian countries and AIDS in Africa compared with the USA).

# 7. Conclusions

## 7.1. KEY FINDINGS

The risk assessment was successful in terms of achieving its initial objectives In this regard the key findings were as follows:

- The utilization of the framework and parameters for the *V. parahaemolyticus* risk assessment facilitated the development of the *V. vulnificus* risk assessment. This essentially ensured that it was possible to develop this risk assessment and also highlighted how existing risk assessments can be adapted and incorporated into new work which involved either the same commodity or possibly also the same pathogen.
- Where additional data were available it was possible to validate certain aspects of the risk assessment model. The exposure assessment predictions were validated by their close agreement with retail study data.
- In the absence of specific dose-response data it was possible to develop a dose-response relationship from exposure predictions and the reported frequency of illness which was effective for risk characterization and the evaluation of interventions.

## 7.2. LIMITATIONS AND CAVEATS

As identified in earlier sections various assumptions had to be made in the course of developing this risk assessment and the lack of data in certain areas means that there are certain limitations to the final risk assessment, which need to be taken into consideration when using the outputs of this work. However, the risk assessment model has been developed such that, as new data become available or countries collect information specific to their situation, these can be incorporated into the risk assessment. The main limitations and caveats that have been identified are outlined below.

In terms of applying this risk assessment to other geographical there are a numbers of issues which need to be specifically considered and perhaps adjusted to take into account the local situation.

- The *V. vulnificus*-temperature relationship in oysters at harvest may not be applicable to other regions or countries with different environmental conditions, such as high salinity.
- Countries harvesting different species of oysters, and that have different post-harvest handling practices or consumption patterns, may have to adjust the model inputs to account for these differences.
- The proportion of susceptible individuals may be very different in some countries, such as those in Asia and Africa that have high prevalence of hepatitis C and HIV/AIDS, respectively, or in countries with high rates of alcoholism.

Some general limitations to this risk assessment were also identified. These were primarily linked to data limitations and the availability of additional data in the future may mean that certain aspects of the risk assessment would need to be revised.

- The dose-response relationship is based on predicted exposure and was sensitive to the different data sources used for exposure assessment. In the current risk assessment, data from two studies (Motes et al., 1998; Tamplin, 1994) were evaluated. Pooling of the data sets resulted in a substantially higher predicted mean *V. vulnificus*/g compared with that obtained based on the Motes et al. data alone. This discrepancy in predictions was found to be a consequence of the higher residual variation of $\log_{10}$ *V. vulnificus* levels in the Tamplin data compared with Motes et al. data, even though the mean $\log_{10}$ *V. vulnificus*/g versus water temperature relationships were comparable. The resulting differences in dose-response and the impact on the evaluation of effectiveness of targeted mitigation levels were appreciable. Use of the Motes et al. data resulted in a more conservative estimate (e.g. slightly higher illness rates) than use of the pooled Motes et al. and Tamplin data sets. When only the Motes et al. data were used, the predicted annual illnesses at targeted mitigation levels of 3 MPN/g and 30 MPN/g were 0.16 and 1.2, respectively. When the Motes et al. and Tamplin data were pooled, the resulting predictions of illnesses at 3 MPN/g and 30 MPN/g decreased to 0.06 and 0.5, respectively. Thus, risk assessors are advised to use caution when pooling data sets and consider the sensitivity of predictions to alternative data sources when evaluating the potential effectiveness of proposed mitigations in reducing illnesses. In this case, predictions based on the Motes et al. data alone appeared to be more in line with independent data on *V. vulnificus*/g at retail, and hence were considered a more appropriate basis for dose-response assessment.
- The dose-response assessment and risk characterization was based on the assumption that all strains are equally virulent and there are no seasonal or regional changes in virulence.

## 7.3. CONCLUSION

The approach of extending the models developed in the FDA-VPRA and FAO/WHO-VPRA to model another pathogen, *V. vulnificus*, greatly facilitated the risk assessment process. The same framework and many of the model inputs were applicable for modelling *V. vulnificus* risk in USA oysters and sufficient data was available to conduct a useful risk assessment. It was also possible to develop the model in such a way as to evaluate the potential effectiveness of various mitigation strategies in terms of reducing *V. vulnificus* levels in oysters, and ultimately reducing the risk of illness.

This model provides a strong basis for countries wanting to undertake a risk assessment on *V. vulnificus* in oysters. However, in order to apply the model it would be important to have data relevant to that country, particularly on *V. vulnificus* numbers in seafood's associated with primary septicaemia, at harvest and the point of consumption, and to characterize the susceptible population within that country. For seafood's other than raw oysters the model would need to be altered and evaluated, although the dose-response data may be applicable to other countries.

The risk assessment also identified a number of issues which require further discussion at a scientific level or are areas for further research. Further resolution of some of these issues may lead to the need for revision of certain aspects of the risk assessment. While it is recognized that having good data on which to base every input to the risk assessment is practically impossible it is also appreciated that a risk assessment is not definitive and should be amenable to updating and revision, as appropriate, as new data and information become available. Ultimately the purpose of a risk assessment is to contribute to the process of decision-making by those responsible for food safety risk management. To be of optimal use for this purpose periodic updating may be necessary. This risk assessment evaluated both past risk management decisions as well as potential risk mitigation strategies thereby allowing risk managers to compare past actions and possible future decisions. While any risk assessment model can only be as good as the data on which it is based, it nevertheless provides a strong visual picture based on the available scientific data of the extent of the risks being faced and how they can be effectively mitigated.

# 8. References

Ama, A.A., Hamdy, M.K. & Toledo, R.T. 1994. Effects of heating, pH and thermoradiation on inactivation of *Vibrio vulnificus*. *Food Microbiology,* **11**: 215–227.

Berlin, D.L., Herson, D.S., Hicks, D.T. & Hoover, D.G. 1999. Response of pathogenic *Vibrio* species to high hydrostatic pressure. *Applied and Environmental Microbiology,* **65**: 2776–2780.

Bisharat, N. & Raz, R. 1997. *Vibrio* infection in Israel due to changes in fish marketing. *Lancet,* **348**: 1585–1586.

Bisharat, N., Agmon, V., Finkelstein, R., Raz, R., Ben-Dror, G., Lemer, L., Soboh, S., Colodner, R., Cameron, D.N., Wykstra, D.L., Swerdlow, D.L. & Farmer III, J.J. 1999. Clinical, epidemiological, and microbiological features of *Vibrio vulnificus* biogroup 3 causing outbreaks of wound infection and bacteraemia in Israel. *Lancet,* **354**: 1424.

Bryan, P.J., Steffan, R.J., DePaola, A., Foster, J.W. & Bej, A.K. 1999. Adaptive response to cold temperatures in *Vibrio vulnificus*. *Current Microbiology,* **38**: 168–175.

Buchanan, R.L., Damert, W.G., Whiting, R.C. & Van Schothorst, M. 1997. Use of epidemiological and food survey data to estimate a purposefully conservative dose-response relationship for *Listeria monocytogenes* levels and incidence of Listeriosis. *Journal of Food Protection,* **60**: 918–922.

Buchanan, R.L., Whiting, R.C. & Damert, W.C. 1997. When is simple good enough: A comparison of the Gompertz, Baranyi, and three-phase linear models for fitting bacterial growth curves. *Food Microbiology,* **14**: 313–326.

CAC [Codex Alimentarius Commission]. 2000. Report of the 33rd Session of the Codex Committee on Food Hygiene. Washington, DC, 23–28 October 2000.

Chuang, Y.C., Yuan, C.Y., Liu, C.Y., Lan, C.K. & Huang, A.H. 1992. *Vibrio vulnificus* infection in Taiwan: report of 28 cases and review of clinical manifestations and treatment. *Clinical Infectious Diseases,* **15**: 271–276.

Cook, D.W. 1994. Effect of time and temperature on multiplication of *Vibrio vulnificus* in postharvest Gulf coast shellstock oysters. *Applied and Environmental Microbiology,* **60**: 3483–3484.

Cook, D.W. 1997a. Refrigeration of oyster shellstock: conditions which minimize the outgrowth of *Vibrio vulnificus*. *Journal of Food Protection,* **60**: 349–352.

Cook, D.W. 1997b. Survey of oysters at first dealer level to assess the effect of the Interstate Shellfish Sanitation Conference's Interim Control Plan to reduce *Vibrio vulnificus* in oysters intended for raw consumption. U.S. Food and Drug Administration.

Cook, D.W. & Ruple, A.D. 1992. Cold storage and mild heat treatment as processing aids to reduce the numbers of *Vibrio vulnificus* in raw oysters. *Journal of Food Protection,* **55**: 985–989.

Cook, D.W., O'Leary, P., Hunsucker, J.C., Sloan, E.M., Bowers, J.C., Blodgett, R.J. & DePaola, A. 2002. *Vibrio vulnificus* and *Vibrio parahaemolyticus* in U.S. retail shell oysters: A national survey June 1998 to July 1999. *Journal of Food Protection,* **65**: 79–87.

Crump, K.S. 1998. On summarizing group exposures in risk assessment: is an arithmetic mean or a geometric mean more appropriate? *Risk Analysis,* **18**(3): 293–297.

Degner, R.L. & Petrone, C. 1994. Consumer and restaurant manager reaction to depurated oysters and clams. Report to the Levy County Board of County Commissioners by the Florida Agricultural Market Research Center, University of Florida.

DePaola, A., Capers, G.M. & Alexander, D. 1994. Densities of *Vibrio vulnificus* in the intestines of fish from the U.S. Gulf Coast. *Applied and Environmental Microbiology,* **60**: 984–988.

DePaola, A., Motes, M.L., Cook, D.W., Veazey, J., Garthright, W.E. & Blodgett, R. 1997. Evaluation of alkaline phosphatase-labeled DNA probe for enumeration of *Vibrio vulnificus* in Gulf Coast oysters. *Journal of Microbiological Methods*, **29**: 115–120.

DePaola, A., Nordstrom, J.L., Dalsgaard, A., Forslund, A., Oliver, J.D., Bates, T., Bourdade, K.L. & Gulig, P.A. 2003. Analysis of *Vibrio vulnificus* from market oysters and septicemia cases for virulence markers. *Applied and Environmental Microbiology,* **69**: 4006–4011.

Desenclos, J.A., Klontz, K.C., Wolfe, L.E. & Hoecheri, S. 1991. The risk of *Vibrio* illness in the Florida raw oyster eating population, 1981–1988. *American Journal of Epidemiology,* **134:** 290–297.

DHHS [U.S. Department of Health and Human Services]. 1999. National Shellfish Sanitation Program Guide for the Control of Molluscan Shellfish. Washington, DC: U.S. Department of Health and Human Services.

FAO/WHO [Food and Agriculture Organization of the United Nations/World Health Organization] (in press). Risk assessment of *Vibrio parahaemolyticus* in seafood's.

FDA [U.S. Food and Drug Administration]. 2001. *Draft Risk Assessment on the Public Health Impacts of Vibrio parahaemolyticus in Raw Molluscan Shellfish*, Washington, DC: U.S. Food and Drug Administration.

Flattery, J. & Bashin B. 2004. A baseline survey of raw oyster consumers in four states, Interstate Shellfish Sanitation Conference (available at http://issc.org/Vibrio_vulnificus_Education/Baseline%20Survey.pdf).

Harris-Young, L., Tamplin, M.L., Fisher, W.S. & Mason, J.W. 1993. Effects of physicochemical factors and bacterial colony morphotype on association of *Vibrio vulnificus* with hemocytes of *Crassostrea virginica. Applied and Environmental Microbiology,* **59**: 1012–1017.

Hlady, G. 1994. Risk assessment and current data: Florida risk assessment and factors associated with risk. pp. 27–33, *in:* W. Watkins and S. McCarthy (eds). Proceedings of the 1994 *Vibrio vulnificus* Workshop. DHHS/FDA/CFSAN, Office of Seafood, Washington, DC, USA.

Hlady, W.G. 1997. *Vibrio* infections associated with raw oyster consumption in Florida, 1981–1994. *Journal of Food Protection,* **60**: 353–357.

Hlady, W.G. & Klontz, K.C. 1996. The Epidemiology of *Vibrio* Infections in Florida, 1983– 1993. *Journal of Infectious Diseases,* **173**: 1176–1180.

Hlady, W.G., Mullen, R.C. & Hopkin, R.S. 1993. *Vibrio vulnificus* from raw oysters. Leading cause of reported deaths from foodborne illness in Florida. *Journal of the Florida Medical Association,* **80**: 536–538.

Jackson, J.K., Murphree, R.L. & Tamplin, M.L. 1997. Evidence that mortality from *Vibrio vulnificus* infection results from single strains among heterogeneous populations in shellfish. *Journal of Clinical Microbiology,* **35**: 2098–2101.

Johnson, D.E., Calia, F.M., Musher, D.M. & Goree, A. 1984. Resistance of *Vibrio vulnificus* to serum bactericidal and opsonizing factors: relation to virulence in suckling mice and humans. *Journal of Infectious Diseases,* **150**: 413–418.

Kaspar, C.W. & Tamplin, M.L. 1993. Effects of temperature and salinity on the survival of *Vibrio vulnificus* in seawater and shellfish. *Applied and Environmental Microbiology,* **59**: 2425–2429.

Kaysner, C.A., Abeyta, C.J.R., Wekell, M.M., DePaola, A., Stott, R.F. & Leitch, J.M. 1987. Virulent strains of *Vibrio vulnificus* isolated from estuaries of the United States West coast. *Applied and Environmental Microbiology,* **53**: 1349–1351.

Kelly, M.T. 1982. Effect of temperature and salinity on *Vibrio (Beneckea) vulnificus* occurrence in a Gulf coast environment. *Applied and Environmental Microbiology,* **44**: 820–824.

Kim, M.S. & Jeong, H.D. 2001. Development of 16S rRNA targeted PCR methods for the detection and differentiation of *Vibrio vulnificus* in marine environments. *Aquaculture,* **193**: 199–211.

Klontz, K.C. 1997. Estimated number of persons at increased risk for *Vibrio vulnificus* septicemia: Memorandum to Phillip C. Spiller, Director of FDA Office of Seafood. Document is attached here as Appendix E.

Klontz, K.C., Timbo, B., Fein, S. & Levy, A. 1995. Prevalence of selected food consumption and preparation behaviors associated with increased risks of food-borne disease. *Journal of Food Protection*, **58**: 927–930.

Koo, J., Marshall, D.L. & DePaola, A. 2001. Antacid increases survival of *Vibrio vulnificus* and *Vibrio vulnificus* phage in a gastrointestinal model. *Applied and Environmental Microbiology,* **67**: 2895–2902.

McCoubrey, D.J. 1996. Risk of *Vibrio vulnificus* infection following consumption of raw commercially harvested North Island oysters. MPH Thesis. The University of Auckland, New Zealand. 86 p.

McCullagh, P. & Nelder, J.A. 1989. *Generalized linear models*. Monographs on Statistics and Applied Probability, vol. 37. London: Chapman and Hall.

Mead, P.S., Slutsker, L., Dietz, V., McGaig, L.F., Bresee, J.S., Shapiro, C., Griffin, P.M. & Tauxe, R.V. 1999. Food-related illness and death in the United States. *Emerging Infectious Diseases,* **5**: 607–625.

Morris, J.G., Wright, A.C., Simpson, L.M., Wood, P.K., Johnson, D.E. & Oliver, J.D. 1987. Virulence of *Vibrio vulnificus*: association with utilization of transferrin-bound iron, and lack of correlation with levels of cytotoxin or protease production. *FEMS Microbiology Letters,* **40**: 55–59.

Motes, M.L. & DePaola, A. 1996. Offshore suspension relaying to reduce levels of *Vibrio vulnificus* in oysters (*Crassostrea virginica*). *Applied and Environmental Microbiology,* **62**: 3875–3877.

Motes, M.L., DePaola, A., Cook, D.W., Veazey, J.E., Hunsucker, J.C., Garthright, W.E., Blodgett, R.J. & Chirtel, S.J. 1998. Influence of water temperature and salinity on *Vibrio vulnificus* in northern Gulf and Atlantic Coast oysters (*Crassostrea virginica*). *Applied and Environmental Microbiology,* **64**: 1459–1465.

NERRS [National Estuarine Research Reserve System]. 2001. Weeks Bay, AL temperature data (available at www.ocrm.nos.noaa.gov/nerr/welcome.html).

Nilsson, L., Oliver, J.D. & Kjelleberg, S. 1991. Resuscitation of *Vibrio vulnificus* from the viable but nonculturable state. *Journal of Bacteriology,* **173**: 5054–5059.

Nilsson, W.B., Paranjpye, R.N., DePaola, A. & Strom, M.S. 2003. Sequence polymorphism of the 16S rRNA gene of *Vibrio vulnificus* is a possible indicator of strain virulence. *Journal of Clinical Microbiology,* **41**: 442–446.

NMFS [National Marine Fisheries Service]. 1998. Fisheries Data for the United States 1990–1998 (available at www.nmfs.noaa.gov).

NOAA [National Oceanic and Atmospheric Administration]. 1999 and various dates. National Climatic Data Center Global Buoy Data (available at www.ncdc.noaa.gov/oa/ncdc.html).

Oliver, J.D. 1989. *Vibrio vulnificus*. pp. 569–600, *in:* M.P. Doyle (ed). *Foodborne bacterial pathogens*. New York, USA: Marcel Dekker, Inc.

Oliver, J.D. 1995. The viable but non-culturable state in the human pathogen *Vibrio vulnificus*. *FEMS Microbiology Letters,* **133**: 203–208.

Oliver, J.D., Warner, R.A. & Cleland, D.R. 1982. Distribution and ecology of *Vibrio vulnificus* and other lactose-fermenting marine vibrios in coastal waters of the Southeastern United States. *Applied and Environmental Microbiology,* **44**: 1404–1414.

O'Neill, K.R., Jones, S.H. & Grimes, D.J. 1992. Seasonal incidence of *Vibrio vulnificus* in the Great Bay estuary of New Hampshire and Maine. *Applied and Environmental Microbiology,* **58**: 3257–3262.

Ono, M., Inoue, Y. & Yokoyama, M. 2001. [A cluster of *V. vulnificus* infection in Kumamoto Prefecture (in Japanese)]. *Infectious Agents Surveillance Reports,* No. 22.

Oonaka, K., Furuhata, K., Iguchi, K., Hara, M. & Fukuyama, M. 2002. [Basic studies on *Vibrio vulnificus* infection: isolation of *V. vulnificus* from sea water, sea mud, and oysters (in Japanese)]. *Kansenshogaku Zasshi,* **76**: 528–535.

Park, S.D., Shon, H.S. & Joh, N.J. 1991. *Vibrio vulnificus* septicemia in Korea: clinical and epidemiologic findings in seventy patients. *Journal of the American Academy of Dermatology,* **24**: 397–403.

Parvathi A, Kumar, H.S., Karunasagar, I. & Karunasagar, I. 2004. Detection and enumeration of *Vibrio vulnificus* in oysters from two estuaries along the South West Coast of India, using molecular methods. *Applied and Environmental Microbiology,* **70**: 6909–6913.

Poole, M.D. & Oliver, J.D. 1978. Experimental pathogenicity and mortality in ligated ileal loop studies of newly reported halophilic lactose-positive *Vibrio* sp. *Infection and Immunity*, **20**: 126–129.

Reyes, A.L., Johnson, C.H., Spalding, P.B. & Stelma, G.N. Jr. 1987. Oral infectivity of *Vibrio vulnificus* in suckling mice. *Journal of Food Protection,* **50**: 1013–1016.

Rose, J.B., Huq, A. & Lipp, E.K. (eds). 1999. Health, climate and infectious disease: A global perspective. A report from American Academy of Microbiology, based on an American Academy of Microbiology colloquium, Tucson, Arizona, USA, 15–17 October 1999.

Ruple, A.D. & Cook, D.W. 1992. *Vibrio vulnificus* and indicator bacteria in shellstock and commercially processed oysters from the Gulf coast. *Journal of Food Protection,* **59**: 667–671.

Scientific Committee on Veterinary Measures Relating to Public Health. 2001. Opinion of the Scientific Committee on Veterinary Measures Relating to Public Health on *Vibrio vulnificus* and *Vibrio parahaemolyticus* (in raw and undercooked seafood) (adopted on 19–20 September 2001). European Commission, Health & Consumer Protection Directorate-General, Directorate C - Scientific Opinions. 64 pp.

Shapiro, R.L., Altekruse, S., Hutwagner, S., Bishop, R., Hammond, R., Wilson, S., Ray, B., Thompson, S., Tauxe, R.V., Griffin, P.M. & *Vibrio* working group. 1998. The role of Gulf Coast oysters harvested in warmer months in *Vibrio vulnificus* infections in the United States, 1988–1996. *Journal of Infectious Diseases,* **178**: 752–759.

Stelma, G.N. Jr., Reyes, A.L., Peeler, J.T., Johnson, C.H. & Spaulding, P.L. 1992. Virulence characteristics of clinical and environmental isolates of *Vibrio vulnificus*. *Applied and Environmental Microbiology,* **58**: 2776–2782.

Strom, M.S. & Paranjpye, R.N. 2000. Epidemiology and pathogenesis of *Vibrio vulnificus*. *Microbes and Infection,* **2**: 177–188.

Sun, Y. & Oliver, J.D. 1994. Effects of GRAS compounds on natural *Vibrio vulnificus* populations in oysters. *Journal of Food Protection,* **57**: 921–923.

Sun, Y. & Oliver, J.D. 1995. Hot sauce: No elimination of *Vibrio vulnificus* in oysters. *Journal of Food Protection,* **58**: 441–442.

Tamplin, M.L. 1990. The ecology of *Vibrio vulnificus* in *Crassostrea virginica*, Williamsburg, VA: Shellfish Institute of North America/National Shellfish Institute.

Tamplin, M.L. 1994. The seasonal occurrence of *Vibrio vulnificus* in shellfish, seawater, and sediment in United States coastal waters. Final report to Salstonstall-Kennedy Grant Program, US Department of Commerce.

Tamplin, M.L. & Capers, G.M. 1992. Persistence of *Vibrio vulnificus* in tissues of Gulf Coast oysters, *Crassostrea virginica*, exposed to seawater disinfected with UV light. *Applied and Environmental Microbiology,* **58**: 1506–1510.

Tamplin, M.L., Rodrick, G.E., Blake, N.J. & Cuba, T. 1982. Isolation and characterization of *Vibrio vulnificus* from two Florida estuaries. *Applied and Environmental Microbiology,* **44**: 1466–1470.

Thamlikitkul, V. 1990. *Vibrio* bacteremia in Siriraj hospital. *Journal of the Medical Association of Thailand,* **73**: 136–138.

Timbo, B.B., Headrick, M., Klontz, K., Street, D. & Wilcox, T. 1996. Raw shellfish consumption and warning labels: results from the 1993 Texas Behavioral Risk Factor Surveillance System (BRFSS) survey. *Texas Medicine*, November: 52.

Tison, D.L. & Kelly, M.T. 1986. Virulence of *Vibrio vulnificus* strains from marine environments. *Applied and Environmental Microbiology,* **51**: 1004–1006.

USDA/ARS [U.S. Department of Agriculture, Agricultural Research Service]. Various dates. Data from 1989–1992 Continuing Survey of Food Intakes by Individuals, 1989–1992 Diet and Health Knowledge Survey, and technical support databases. National Technical Information Service, Springfield, VA, USA (available at www.ntis.gov).

Vanoy, R.W., Tamplin, M.L. & Schwartz, J.R. 1992. Ecology of *Vibrio vulnificus* in Galveston Bay oysters, suspended particulate matter, sediment and seawater: Detection by monoclonal antibody-immunoassay-most probable number procedures. *Journal of Industrial Microbiology,* **9**: 219–223.

Wright, A.C., Simpson, L.M. & Oliver, J.D. 1981. Role of iron in the pathogenesis of *Vibrio vulnificus* infections. *Infection and Immunity,* **34**: 503–507.

# Appendices

## Appendix A.

# MODEL IMPLEMENTATION

Briefly, in a Monte Carlo simulation approach to quantitative risk assessment, variability distributions and/or quantitative relationships between identified model components (e.g. variables) are estimated based on the available data. Where applicable, uncertainties associated with these estimated distributions and relationships are also quantified. These variability and uncertainty distributions are then coded into simulation software in order to investigate, via simulation, the distributions of model outputs of interest (such as dose and risk associated with mitigations). The term "Monte Carlo" in particular refers to the approach of simulating the output distributions of interest by generating random samples of model inputs and then propagating these sampled values through model-based equations and relationships to obtain corresponding values (or samples) of relevant output distributions. This appendix describes the implementation (i.e. coding) of a model in the selected Monte Carlo simulation software.

The calculations in this assessment were performed primarily using the Monte Carlo simulation software Analytica® (Lumina Decision Systems Inc., USA). However, due to memory limitations of the Analytica® software constraining the performing of a large number of scenarios and/or samples, the month- and year-specific dose calculations used in the dose-response assessment were implemented in @Risk® (Palisade Corporation, USA) and SAS®. In all cases, simulations were conducted with 100 uncertainty samples and a simple random sample of 10 000 with respect to variability factors.

## ANALYTICA® MODEL SIMULATION STRUCTURE FOR RISK ASSESSMENT OF *V. VULNIFICUS* IN RAW OYSTERS

Following the format of the FDA-VPRA and the FAO/WHO-VPRA, the structure of the simulation was organized into three parts: (1) simulation of the distribution of *Vibrio vulnificus* numbers in oysters at the time of harvest; (2) simulation of the effect of post-harvest processing on the distribution of *V. vulnificus* numbers at the point of consumption; and (3) subsequent simulation of the distribution of doses consumed and the corresponding risk according to the inferred dose-response relation.

Specification of the model in Analytica®* was accomplished by specifying "chance" nodes and interrelationships between these nodes in an influence diagram for the simulation. Additional nodes of the influence diagram were used to contain supporting information such as function and index definitions that are referenced in the specification of the chance nodes representing the parameters of the model to be simulated per se. Implementation of uncertainty in the simulation was accomplished by using array indexing. By using this feature of the software, a sequence of 100 simulations (representing different plausible values of the

* A description of the variable names used in the Analytica® model are provided in Table A.1.

uncertainty factors) were performed concurrently in order to obtain summary statistics of the distribution of the relevant output (e.g. dose and risk) over the distribution of uncertainty. An array index was also used to implement season. Thus, parameters that vary according to season (such as duration of harvesting) have different values according to the season index.

Figure A.1 shows the Analytica® influence diagram of the model for harvest density calculations. Water temperature influences $\log_{10}$ *V. vulnificus*/g at harvest, from which the distribution of *V. vulnificus*/g is obtained by taking the antilog. The definition of the water temperature node is:

Normal(Temp_distr[Tempparms='mu'],Temp_distr[Tempparms='sigma'])

The temperature parameter array "Temp_distr" (the "temperature distributions" node) contains a sample of 100 year-to-year variations of mean ("mu") and standard deviation ("sigma") of the day-to-day variability distribution of water temperature. Each element in the array corresponds to a separate simulation so that a sequence of 100 simulations can be obtained once values of parameters are loaded into the array. A separate influence diagram was implemented to obtain samples of 100 year-to-year variations of (correlated) water temperature parameters according to the appropriate uncertainty distribution.

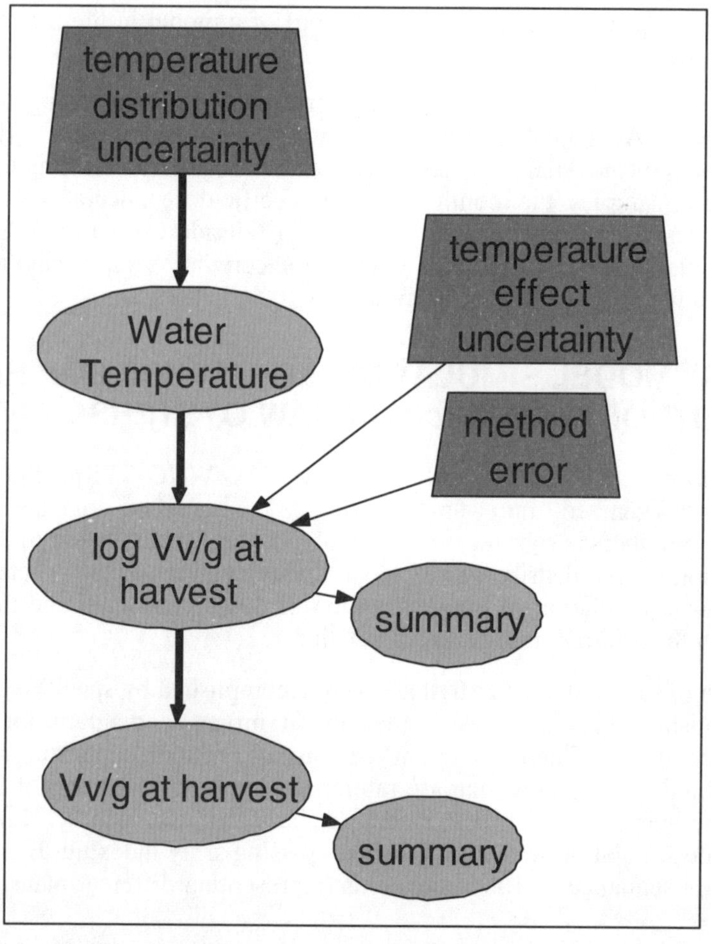


**Figure A.1** Structure of simulation model of *V. vulnificus*/g (*Vv*/g) at harvest.

The definition of the $\log_{10}$ *V. vulnificus*/g at-harvest node is:

min([6,Normal( Temperature_effect_[ T_parm='a']

+Temperature_effect_[ T_parm='b']*Wtemp

+Temperature_effect_[ T_parm='c']*Wtemp*Wtemp,

sqrt(Temperature_effect_[ T_parm='sigma']^2-Method_error_var))])

This is simply the normal distribution of $\log_{10}$ *V. vulnificus*/g at any randomly sampled temperature value ("Wtemp") in accordance with the parameters of the *V. vulnificus* levels versus temperature regression ("Temperature_effect"). Since the estimate of variation of observed levels includes method error, an estimate of method error must be subtracted to obtain an estimate of population variation of true or actual levels. A point estimate of 0.12 for method error variance was assumed in these calculations. Additionally, based on the assumption of a maximum density of $10^6$ *V. vulnificus*/g, the distribution was truncated at 6 logs. The distribution of *V. vulnificus*/g is obtained by taking the antilog of the distribution of $\log_{10}$ *V. vulnificus*/g.

The Analytica® influence diagram for the effect of post-harvest processing is shown in Figure A.2. Water temperature and Air/Water temperature differences define the node representing the variation of ambient temperature of oysters prior to refrigeration. For each Monte Carlo random sample of ambient air temperature, the corresponding growth rate is defined as:

Max(0,0.011*(*Air_temperature*-13))

The chance nodes representing variation of time on the water (length of harvesting operations) and time required to cool oysters down to no-growth conditions (≤13°C) influence the chance nodes for the amount of growth that occurs prior to time of first refrigeration and then subsequently as the oysters cool. These relationships are defined as:

Min( [ Log_vv_g_h + Growth_rate*Time_oysters_unrefr, 6]) - Log_vv_g_h

and

Min( [ Log_vv_g_h+Outgrowth_1+Growth_rate*(Time_to_cool+1)/2, 6] )

- (Log_vv_g_h+Outgrowth_1)

The variable "*Log_vv_g_h*" here represents the density per g at harvest (from the previous influence diagram). "*Outgrowth_1*" is the number of logs of growth occurring prior to first refrigeration if oysters are unrefrigerated for a period defined by "*Time_oysters_unrefr*". However, no growth is permitted that would raise numbers above 6 $\log_{10}$. Similarly, the latter equation defines the extent of growth during cool down duration ("*Time_to_cool*"), subject to a restriction that no growth is allowed that would raise numbers above 6 $\log_{10}$.

The final output parameter in the influence diagram is the density at consumption:

Log_vv_g_h + Outgrowth_1 + Outgrowth_2 - Die_off_during_stor

The overall effect of these calculations is that simulated samples of density at harvest are adjusted upward by the distributions of extent of growth prior to and during refrigeration.

Then the resulting distribution is adjusted down by the effect of random extent of die-off as a consequence of random duration of storage of from 1 to 21 days.

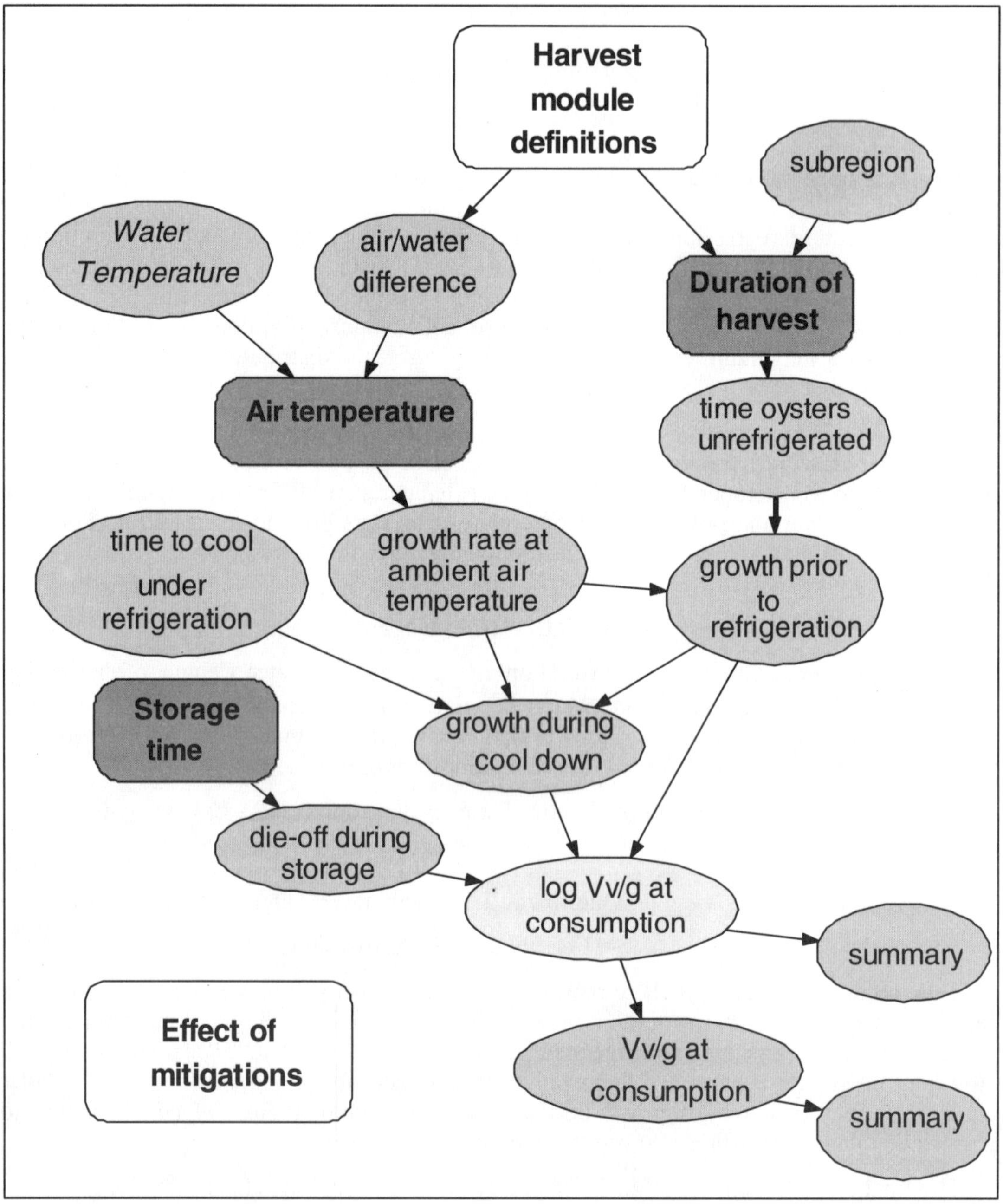


**Figure A.2** Structure of simulation model of effect of post-harvest handling on *V. vulnificus*/g (*Vv*/g) density.

The third and final component of the model is the simulation of the distribution of doses consumed and the resulting distribution of risk. The structure of these calculations is shown in Figure A.3. As shown, and following the structure of the FDA-VPRA and the FAO/WHO VPRA, the distribution of the serving size is obtained by combining the distribution of the number of oysters consumed with the distribution of the average weight (grams) per oyster. This distribution is then combined with the distribution of *V. vulnificus*/g at consumption to obtain the dose distribution.

At this point, the simulation is structured to calculate the mean risk corresponding to each simulated mean dose, where the mean is taken with respect to variability factors for each of the 100 combinations of uncertainty factor samples. The effect of dose-response on risk was not imbedded at the level of individual doses because it was observed that this was inappropriate as a consequence of the apparent effects of aggregation bias (see Appendix C). The dose-response used in the assessment was obtained by fitting a dose-response model to (inferred) data points representing mean risk versus mean dose consumed over a relatively large number of servings. Depending upon the nature of the relationship between risk and dose on the individual level and characteristics (e.g. skew ness) of the distribution of dose, the relationship of mean risk versus mean dose is not equal to the relationship between risk and dose on the level of the individual. This was found to be the case in the present assessment and, consequently, the inferred dose-response relationship obtained by correlation of mean dose reconstruction versus mean risk was not taken to apply on the individual level (e.g. with respect to simulated individual doses according to variability factors).

The effect of mitigations was simulated by altering the parameter definitions corresponding to the baseline assessment and then re-running the simulation to obtain simulation-based estimates of the effect on the risk. Three sets of mitigations affecting levels of *V. vulnificus* were considered here. First, regardless of the method used to reduce levels of *V. vulnificus* to standards of 3/g, 30/g and 300/g, the risk associated with these mean levels was calculated. The distribution of $\log_{10}$ *V. vulnificus*/g was calculated for each target level (3/g, 30/g and 300/g) by assuming that the variance of $\log_{10}$ *V. vulnificus*/g at time of consumption was unaffected by the mitigation and that only the mean $\log_{10}$ *V. vulnificus*/g was reduced in a manner that achieved the specified standard for mean *V. vulnificus*/g. This reduction was applied to all simulated samples of *V. vulnificus*/g at consumption. If *V. vulnificus*/g at consumption was already less than the standard, as may commonly be the case in the winter, then the mitigation was assumed to have no effect. The resulting distribution of *V. vulnificus*/g was then combined with the distribution of grams consumed and dose-response relation to obtain mean risk per serving and annual number of cases, along with attendant uncertainties.

The effect of time unrefrigerated and the implementation of the 1996 ISSC reductions in time-to-refrigeration were obtained by fixing the time unrefrigerated to either fixed non-varying levels or to a distribution of values inferred to correspond to pre-1996 harvesting practices in the USA Gulf Coast.

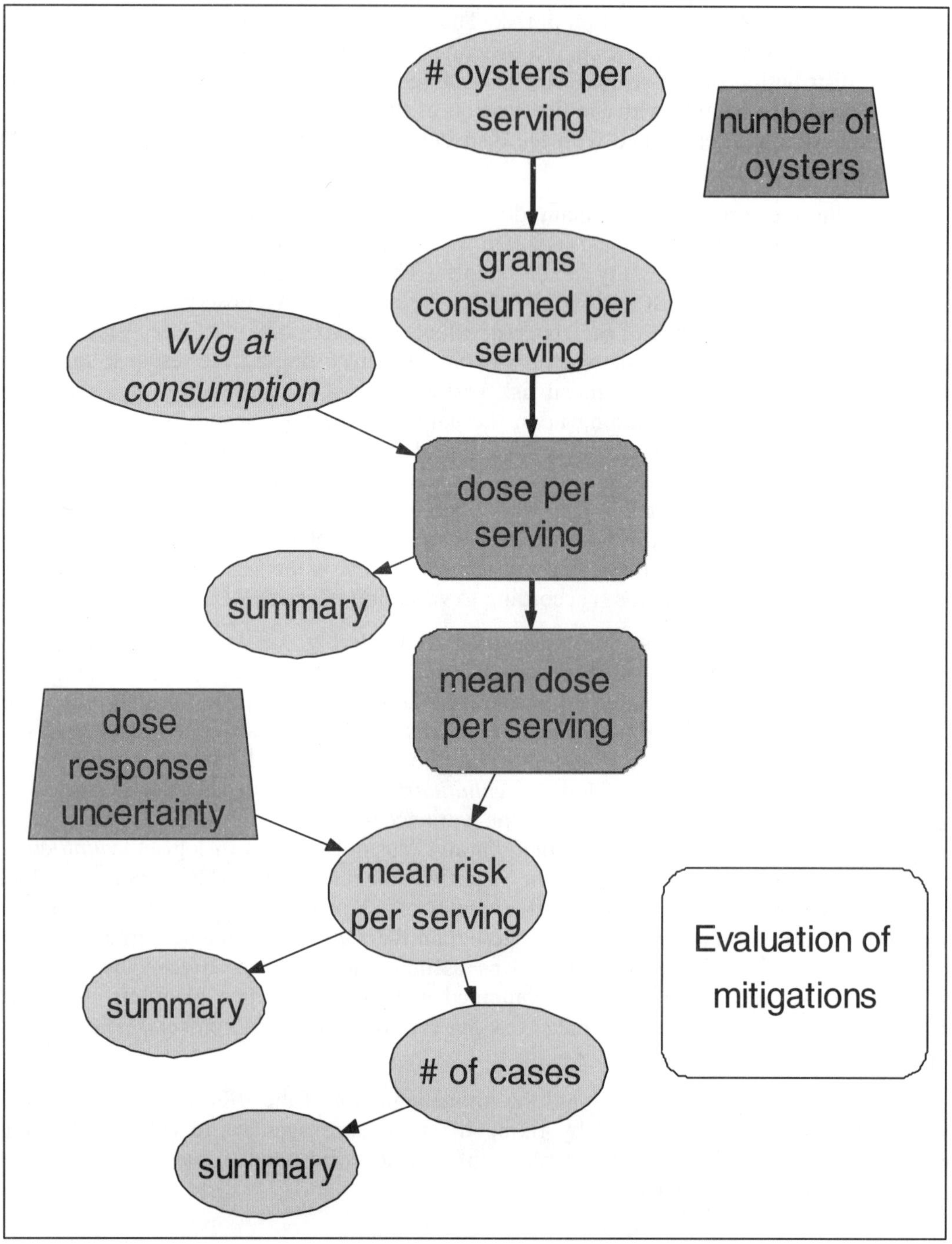


**Figure A.3** Structure of simulation model of distribution of dose of *V. vulnificus* (*Vv*/g) consumed and resulting distribution of risk.

**Table A.1.** Description of the variable names used in the Analytica® model

| Analytica® variable names | Description |
|---|---|
| Temp_distr | uncertainty/variability of parameters of the distribution of water temperature |
| Temperature_effect | uncertainty of the parameters of the $\log_{10}$ *V. vulnificus*/g versus water temperature relationship |
| Wtemp | water temperature at time of harvest |
| Log_vv_g_h | $\log_{10}$ *V. vulnificus*/g at time of harvest |
| Vv_g_h | *V. vulnificus*/g at time of harvest |
| Air_temperature | air temperature at time of harvest |
| Duration_of_harvest | length of harvesting (e.g., dredging) operations |
| Time_oysters_unrefr | time from collection (e.g. dredging) until placed under refrigeration |
| Growth_rate | growth rate while held at ambient air temperature prior to refrigeration |
| Outgrowth_1 | amount of growth from time of harvest to time placed under refrigeration |
| Time_to_cool | length of time to reach no growth temperature once under refrigeration |
| Outgrowth_2 | amount of growth occurring after placed under refrigeration |
| Storage_time | length of time of cold storage prior to consumption |
| Die_off_during_stor | $\log_{10}$ reduction of *V. vulnificus*/g during cold storage |
| Log_vv_g_r | $\log_{10}$ *V. vulnificus*/g at time of consumption |
| Vv_g_r | *V. vulnificus*/g at time of consumption |
| Num_oysters | number of oysters per serving |
| Amount_consumed | gram weight of oysters per serving |
| Total_vv_ingested | number of *V. vulnificus* ingested per serving |
| Mean_vv_ingested | mean number of *V. vulnificus* ingested per serving |
| Dose_response_uncert | uncertainty of parameters of the dose-response relationship |
| Risk_per_serving | mean risk per serving |
| Ncases | number of reported cases predicted |

## Appendix B.

# ESTIMATED MODEL PARAMETERS IN THE EXPOSURE ASSESSMENT

Many of the model parameters used in the present assessment were obtained from the FDA-VPRA and FAO/WHO-VPRA (e.g. water/air temperatures, distribution of time unrefrigerated). However, *V. vulnificus*-specific estimates of levels versus water temperature at time of harvest and point estimates of parameters such as method error, growth rates and die-off rates during cold storage, were substituted for the corresponding *V. parahaemolyticus*-specific estimates. Additionally, given an identified uncertainty as to appropriate prediction of temperature effects on at-harvest levels due to conflicting sources of information (different data sets), the sensitivity of the risk assessment to this uncertainty was evaluated by performing replicate analyses with different estimates of the temperature relationship. This relationship underlies both the risk characterization and the dose-response assessment.

## Water temperature

Water temperatures used for baseline risk assessment and risk characterization were taken to have a year-to-year and seasonal distribution as specified in the FDA-VPRA and FAO/WHO-VPRA.

However, given that the dose-response assessment was conducted by reconstructing estimated mean doses consumed for each month in the period between 1995 and 2001 (corresponding to the period for which case data was available), the temperature data from the NOAA NBDC measurement buoy at Dauphin Island, Alabama, USA, was supplemented with data from the NERRS site at Weeks Bay, Alabama, USA, and these data were then analysed on a month- and year-specific basis for later use in simulations using @Risk® and SAS® software for the dose reconstruction prior to the dose-response assessment per se. The results of the analysis of these water temperature data is given in Table B.1. Monthly averages over the 1995–2001 period are shown in Table B.2.

## $Log_{10}$ *V. vulnificus/g* versus water temperature

Two data sets were identified to estimate and characterize the relationship between *V. vulnificus/g* and water temperature at the time of harvest. Ostensibly, basing the assessment on estimates from these different data sets or basing the assessment on estimates after pooling the data results in different implications for low-dose risk (e.g. at 3/g, 30/g or 300/g mitigation standards). Consequently, to investigate the sensitivity of the results of the assessment to these different approaches, model simulations were conducted for four alternatives: (1) Motes et al. (1998) data alone (with unaveraged replicate samples considered separate samples); (2) Motes et al. data alone (with average of replicate samples considered a single observation); (3) Tamplin data alone; and (4) pooled data of Tamplin and Motes et al. (unaveraged replicate data considered as separate observations).

**Table B.1** Estimates of month- and year-specific mean and standard deviation of day-to-day water temperature variation (Dauphin Island and Weeks Bay, Alabama, USA; data for 1995–2001).

| Month and year | Mean water temperature | Std deviation of day-to-day variations in water temperature | Mean air-water temperature difference | Std deviation of day-to-day variations in air-water temperature difference | Data source |
|---|---|---|---|---|---|
| Jan-95 | 12.41 | 1.55 | -0.46 | 3.16 | DPIA average 1995–2001 |
| Feb-95 | 13.74 | 1.70 | -0.45 | 2.95 | |
| Mar-95 | 16.66 | 2.15 | -0.62 | 2.59 | |
| Apr-95 | 20.49 | 1.90 | -1.11 | 2.14 | |
| May-95 | 25.08 | 1.84 | -1.22 | 1.34 | |
| Jun-95 | 28.19 | 1.36 | -1.28 | 1.14 | |
| Jul-95 | 29.46 | 1.03 | -1.18 | 1.25 | |
| Aug-95 | 29.75 | 0.97 | -1.65 | 1.09 | |
| Sep-95 | 28.38 | 1.72 | -1.95 | 1.21 | |
| Oct-95 | 20.99 | 1.99 | -1.54 | 2.01 | Weeks Bay |
| Nov-95 | 17.49 | 1.87 | -1.48 | 2.94 | Weeks Bay |
| Dec-95 | 13.37 | 4.52 | -1.07 | 3.56 | Weeks Bay |
| Jan-96 | 11.63 | 2.28 | -0.46 | 3.16 | Weeks Bay |
| Feb-96 | 13.75 | 4.88 | -0.45 | 2.95 | Weeks Bay |
| Mar-96 | 15.62 | 3.08 | -0.62 | 2.59 | Weeks Bay |
| Apr-96 | 22.88 | 1.15 | -2.06 | 2.43 | DPIA |
| May-96 | 26.35 | 2.24 | -1.44 | 1.01 | DPIA |
| Jun-96 | 28.58 | 1.66 | -1.35 | 0.96 | DPIA |
| Jul-96 | 30.05 | 0.75 | -1.27 | 1.09 | DPIA |
| Aug-96 | 29.66 | 0.52 | -2.05 | 0.89 | DPIA |
| Sep-96 | 28.56 | 1.20 | -1.72 | 1.27 | DPIA |
| Oct-96 | 22.42 | 1.51 | -1.52 | 2.15 | DPIA |
| Nov-96 | 18.00 | 2.09 | -1.22 | 3.39 | DPIA |
| Dec-96 | 13.99 | 2.75 | +0.13 | 4.60 | DPIA |
| Jan-97 | 12.93 | 4.13 | -0.46 | 3.16 | Weeks Bay |
| Feb-97 | 13.62 | 1.80 | -0.46 | 3.24 | DPIA |
| Mar-97 | 18.71 | 1.62 | -0.23 | 1.91 | DPIA |
| Apr-97 | 19.21 | 1.16 | -1.05 | 2.21 | DPIA |
| May-97 | 24.26 | 2.10 | -1.34 | 1.35 | DPIA |
| Jun-97 | 27.18 | 1.52 | -1.63 | 1.43 | DPIA |
| Jul-97 | 29.35 | 1.78 | -1.00 | 1.52 | DPIA |
| Aug-97 | 29.42 | 1.45 | -1.30 | 1.08 | DPIA |
| Sep-97 | 28.85 | 1.20 | -1.89 | 1.00 | DPIA |
| Oct-97 | 22.76 | 3.51 | -1.84 | 2.47 | DPIA |
| Nov-97 | 16.35 | 1.67 | -1.49 | 2.64 | DPIA |
| Dec-97 | 13.33 | 2.36 | -1.49 | 3.42 | DPIA |
| Jan-98 | 12.93 | 1.16 | +0.26 | 2.78 | DPIA |
| Feb-98 | 13.49 | 1.85 | +0.08 | 1.73 | DPIA |
| Mar-98 | 15.19 | 2.27 | -0.77 | 3.38 | DPIA |
| Apr-98 | 20.52 | 0.99 | -1.18 | 1.93 | DPIA |
| May-98 | 26.23 | 2.13 | -0.62 | 1.13 | DPIA |
| Jun-98 | 29.06 | 2.00 | -1.05 | 1.09 | DPIA |
| Jul-98 | 29.97 | 1.65 | -0.93 | 1.58 | DPIA |
| Aug-98 | 30.77 | 0.92 | -1.46 | 0.88 | DPIA |
| Sep-98 | 27.70 | 1.17 | -1.20 | 1.14 | DPIA |

| Month and year | Mean water temperature | Std deviation of day-to-day variations in water temperature | Mean air-water temperature difference | Std deviation of day-to-day variations in air-water temperature difference | Data source |
|---|---|---|---|---|---|
| Oct-98 | 24.06 | 2.68 | -1.28 | 1.56 | DPIA |
| Nov-98 | 21.78 | 4.03 | -2.46 | 2.14 | DPIA |
| Dec-98 | 23.74 | 1.40 | -1.07 | 3.56 | Weeks Bay |
| Jan-99 | 15.07 | 3.93 | -0.46 | 3.16 | Weeks Bay |
| Feb-99 | 17.19 | 2.78 | -0.45 | 2.95 | Weeks Bay |
| Mar-99 | 17.58 | 1.23 | -0.62 | 2.59 | Weeks Bay |
| Apr-99 | 24.13 | 2.37 | -1.11 | 2.14 | Weeks Bay |
| May-99 | 25.17 | 1.51 | -1.22 | 1.34 | Weeks Bay |
| Jun-99 | 29.29 | 0.81 | -1.28 | 1.14 | Weeks Bay |
| Jul-99 | 30.00 | 1.25 | -1.18 | 1.25 | Weeks Bay |
| Aug-99 | 31.95 | 1.17 | -1.65 | 1.09 | Weeks Bay |
| Sep-99 | 27.49 | 2.21 | -1.95 | 1.21 | Weeks Bay |
| Oct-99 | 23.52 | 2.60 | -1.54 | 2.01 | Weeks Bay |
| Nov-99 | 19.49 | 1.96 | -1.48 | 2.94 | Weeks Bay |
| Dec-99 | 15.84 | 1.88 | -1.07 | 3.56 | Weeks Bay |
| Jan-00 | 14.74 | 3.53 | -0.46 | 3.16 | Weeks Bay |
| Feb-00 | 16.76 | 3.38 | -0.45 | 2.95 | Weeks Bay |
| Mar-00 | 21.57 | 0.87 | -0.62 | 2.59 | Weeks Bay |
| Apr-00 | 22.30 | 1.79 | -1.11 | 2.14 | Weeks Bay |
| May-00 | 27.75 | 1.68 | -1.22 | 1.34 | Weeks Bay |
| Jun-00 | 30.10 | 1.12 | -1.28 | 1.14 | Weeks Bay |
| Jul-00 | 31.58 | 1.05 | -1.18 | 1.25 | Weeks Bay |
| Aug-00 | 31.10 | 1.21 | -1.65 | 1.09 | Weeks Bay |
| Sep-00 | 27.83 | 2.62 | -1.95 | 1.21 | Weeks Bay |
| Oct-00 | 22.58 | 3.49 | -1.54 | 2.01 | Weeks Bay |
| Nov-00 | 18.13 | 5.23 | -1.48 | 2.94 | Weeks Bay |
| Dec-00 | 12.75 | 2.41 | -1.07 | 3.56 | Weeks Bay |
| Jan-01 | 10.53 | 3.47 | -0.46 | 3.16 | Weeks Bay |
| Feb-01 | 17.10 | 3.04 | -0.45 | 2.95 | Weeks Bay |
| Mar-01 | 16.81 | 3.07 | -0.62 | 2.59 | Weeks Bay |
| Apr-01 | 22.34 | 2.79 | -1.11 | 2.14 | Weeks Bay |
| May-01 | 25.93 | 1.96 | -1.22 | 1.34 | Weeks Bay |
| Jun-01 | 29.28 | 1.26 | -1.28 | 1.14 | Weeks Bay |
| Jul-01 | 29.46 | 1.03 | -1.18 | 1.25 | DPIA average 1995–2001 |
| Aug-01 | 29.75 | 0.97 | -1.65 | 1.09 | |
| Sep-01 | 28.38 | 1.72 | -1.95 | 1.21 | |
| Oct-01 | 22.37 | 2.18 | -1.54 | 2.01 | |
| Nov-01 | 17.78 | 2.42 | -1.48 | 2.94 | |
| Dec-01 | 14.86 | 2.04 | -1.07 | 3.56 | |

NOTE: Air-water temperature differences are always DPIA [Dauphin Island, Alabama] (average or month-specific) since no air temperature measurements are available for Weeks Bay.

**Table B.2** Estimates of monthly mean and standard deviation of day-to-day water temperature variation (Dauphin Island and Weeks Bay, Alabama, USA; data for 1995–2001).

| Month | Mean water temperature (°C) | Standard deviation of day-to-day variations in water temperature | Mean air-water temperature difference | Standard deviation of day-to-day variations in air-water temperature difference |
|---|---|---|---|---|
| Jan | 12.89 | 2.86 | -0.35 | 3.11 |
| Feb | 15.09 | 2.78 | -0.37 | 2.82 |
| Mar | 17.45 | 2.04 | -0.58 | 2.60 |
| Apr | 21.70 | 1.74 | -1.25 | 2.16 |
| May | 25.82 | 1.92 | -1.18 | 1.26 |
| Jun | 28.81 | 1.39 | -1.31 | 1.15 |
| Jul | 29.98 | 1.22 | -1.13 | 1.31 |
| Aug | 30.34 | 1.03 | -1.63 | 1.03 |
| Sep | 28.17 | 1.69 | -1.80 | 1.18 |
| Oct | 22.67 | 2.56 | -1.54 | 2.03 |
| Nov | 18.43 | 2.75 | -1.58 | 2.85 |
| Dec | 15.41 | 2.48 | -0.96 | 3.69 |

The results of censored regression analysis to obtain estimates of the *V. vulnificus/g* versus water temperature relationship are given in Tables B.3 and B.4. The resulting maximum likelihood estimates of median and mean *V. vulnificus*/g versus water temperature are shown in Figures B.1 and B.2 for comparison. The mean levels versus water temperature are based on estimates of population variation in log levels after subtracting the effect of method error on residual variation. It is important to note that the difference between Motes et al. and the Tamplin-based estimates includes differences in the estimates of the residual about the regression. Mean levels versus water temperature are influenced by both differences in median levels versus water temperature and differences in estimates of population variation.

**Table B.3** Maximum Likelihood Estimates (MLEs) of *V. vulnificus/g* versus water temperature relationship.

| Study | No. of samples | $\alpha$ | $\beta$ | $\gamma$ | $\sigma$ |
|---|---|---|---|---|---|
| Motes et al. (unaveraged) | 309 | -6.06051 | 0.587563 | -0.00915 | 0.815649 |
| Motes et al. (averaged replicates) | 156 | -5.65727 | 0.558317 | -0.00862 | 0.731404 |
| Tamplin | 188 | -8.54286 | 0.668044 | -0.0088 | 1.386536 |
| Pooled data (Motes + Tamplin) | 507 | -6.88271 | 0.60296 | -0.00865 | 1.063787 |

NOTES: (1) The regression model was: mean $\log_{10}$ (*V. vulnificus/g*) = $\alpha + \beta$*WTEMP + $\gamma$*WTEMP$^2$; standard deviation of observed $\log_{10}$ (*V. vulnificus/g*) = $\sigma$. Data sets used are those of Motes et al., 1998, and Tamplin et al., 1982.

**Table B.4** Uncertainty estimates of *V. vulnificus*/g versus water temperature relationship (Variance-covariance matrix of parameter estimates).

| Study | | α | β | γ | σ |
|---|---|---|---|---|---|
| Motes et al. | α | 0.651448 | -0.05859 | 0.00125 | -0.00075 |
| (unaveraged) | β | -0.05859 | 0.005421 | -0.00012 | 5.55E-05 |
| | γ | 0.00125 | -0.00012 | 2.6E-06 | -1E-06 |
| | σ | -0.00075 | 5.55E-05 | -1E-06 | 0.001138 |
| Motes et al. | α | 1.028017 | -0.0925775 | 0.0019772 | -0.0006617 |
| (averaged replicates) | β | -0.092577 | 0.0085767 | -0.0001867 | 0.0000523 |
| | γ | 0.001977 | -0.0001867 | 0.0000041 | -0.0000010 |
| | σ | -0.000661 | 0.0000523 | -0.0000010 | 0.0017459 |
| Tamplin | α | 3.296018 | -0.29773 | 0.006407 | -0.01757 |
| | β | -0.29773 | 0.027519 | -0.0006 | 0.001278 |
| | γ | 0.006407 | -0.0006 | 1.34E-05 | -2.3E-05 |
| | σ | -0.01757 | 0.001278 | -2.3E-05 | 0.006634 |
| Pooled data | α | 0.6913 | -0.06237 | 1.34E-03 | -1.83E-03 |
| (Motes + Tamplin) | β | -0.06237 | 5.77E-03 | -1.26E-04 | 1.32E-04 |
| | γ | 1.34E-03 | -1.26E-04 | 2.78E-06 | -2.35E-06 |
| | σ | -1.83E-03 | 1.32E-04 | -2.35E-06 | 1.30E-03 |

NOTES: (1) The regression model was: mean $\log_{10}$ (*V. vulnificus/g*) = $\alpha + \beta$*WTEMP + $\gamma$*WTEMP$^2$; standard deviation of observed $\log_{10}$ (*V. vulnificus/g*) = $\sigma$. Data sets used are those of Motes et al., 1998, and Tamplin et al., 1982.

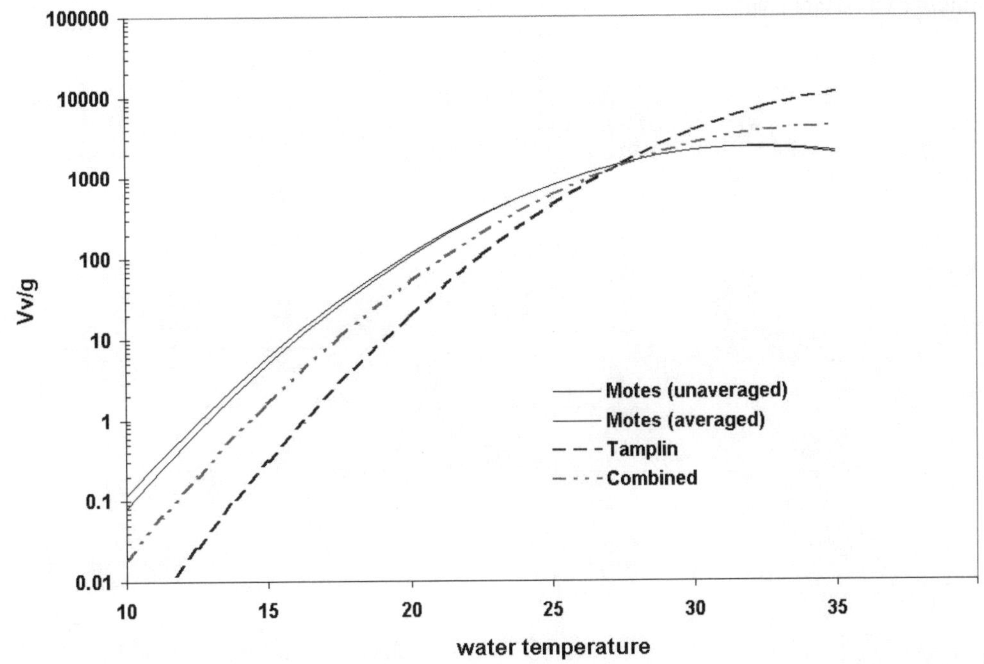


**Figure B.1** Maximum Likelihood Estimates (MLEs) of median *V. vulnificus*/g (Vv/g) versus water temperature (°C) relationship.

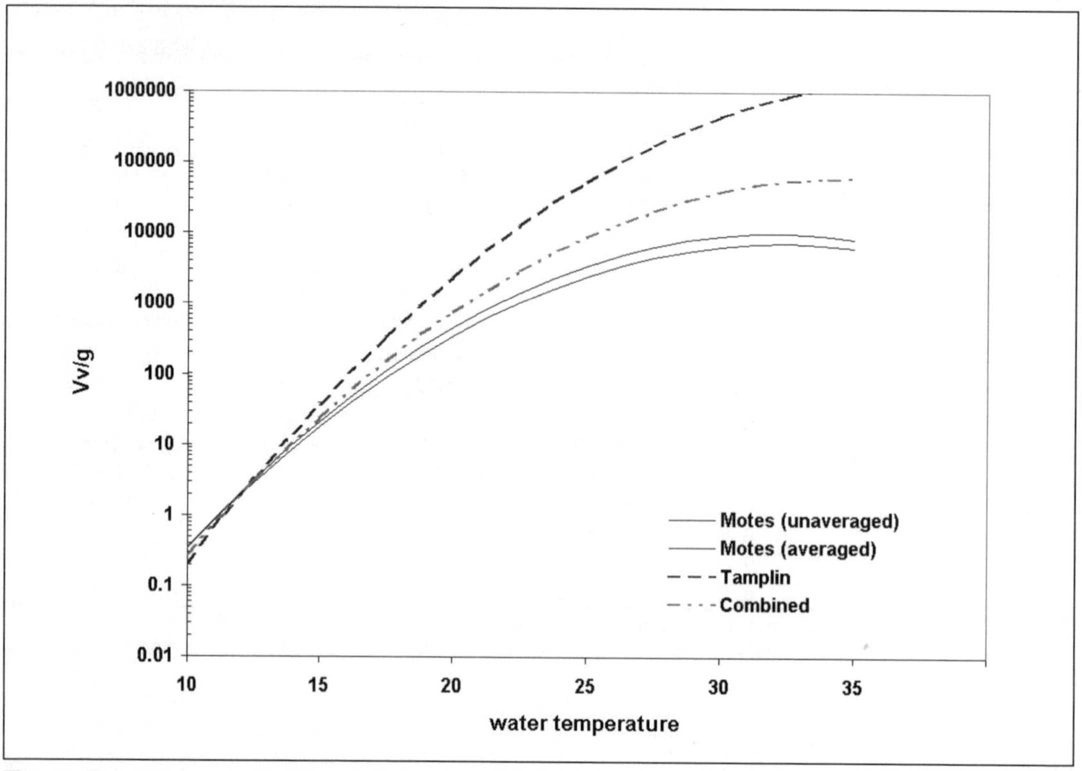


**Figure B.2** Maximum Likelihood Estimates (MLEs) of mean *V. vulnificus*/g (Vv/g) versus water temperature (°C) relationship.

# Appendix C.

# DOSE-RESPONSE ASSESSMENT

The dose-response assessment approach utilized in this assessment is a synthesis of the epidemiological data with dose reconstruction. Dose reconstruction must be performed in the present context because there is (typically) no case-specific information on dose captured along with other attributes of the epidemiological cases reported to surveillance systems. In essence, the true doses associated with illnesses are lost or "missing" and so dose reconstruction is necessary. Similarly, the true doses associated with the large number of eating occasions that did not lead to illness are also missing. This contrasts sharply with a dose-response assessment based on feeding trials with human volunteers, where, by definition, the dose administered is known (up to Poisson variation in the delivery vehicle or inoculum).

Although the actual doses associated with reported illnesses are not known, a reasonable estimate of a dose-response can be obtained if dose reconstruction is feasible and a suitable estimate is available of the number of at-risk servings (or eating occasions). For the present assessment, month- and year-specific water temperature was identified. Based on these data, month- and year-specific dose distributions can be derived based on the modelling approach developed to predict the dose distribution as a consequence of temperature. Reconstruction of the dose distribution can be based on any one of several reasonable partitions of the seasonality of water temperatures, *V. vulnificus* densities and number of cases occurring (e.g. monthly versus seasonal partition). For the present assessment, a partitioning by month was adopted. The observed month- and year-specific oyster-related USA case data is shown in Table C.1.

Given a reconstructed or inferred set of dose distributions and the number of cases occurring, the only remaining information needed is an estimate of the number of at-risk servings. For the present assessment, this was obtained from oyster landings data, summarized on a month-by-month basis. Dividing the number of cases observed (in a given month) by the number of serving provides an estimate of the mean risk per serving for that month. It should be recognized that, within any given month, there is a distribution of risk per serving and that the mean risk is but one characteristic of this distribution.

A dose-response can be estimated by fitting a parametric model to the inferred mean risk versus an appropriate summary measure of the reconstructed dose distributions. What summary statistic of the dose distribution is most appropriate depends on the assumed dose-response relation being fitted to the data. When the dose-response is convex, it has been shown that the arithmetic mean is a more appropriate summary statistic of the dose distribution than the geometric mean (Crump, 1998). When the dose-response relation is concave, the arithmetic mean of the dose distribution is still frequently preferable (Crump, 1998). Two dose-response models commonly used in microbial risk assessment, the Beta-Poisson and the Exponential, are both concave functions of dose. Both of these models were considered in the current assessment and, following Crump, the arithmetic mean of the dose distribution (for each grouping or partitioning of the data) was considered to be the appropriate summary measure of the distribution.

It is important to recognize that, whatever summary measure of the dose distribution is used, the result of fit of a model to data points representing summary statistics of risk versus dose distributions is not necessarily a model of individual-level risk versus individual-level dose. This is a consequence of the possibility of aggregation bias, which is discussed extensively in the epidemiological literature (Piantadosi, Byar and Green, 1988; Greenland and Morgenstern, 1989; Richardson, Stucker and Hemon, 1987). From aggregate-level data, estimating the relationship between exposure and risk at the individual level can be problematical.

Based on all of these considerations, the dose-response assessment for *V. vulnificus* was conducted by reconstructing the dose distributions corresponding to month- and year-specific temperature parameters using each of 3 identified data source alternatives (Motes et al., Tamplin, and combined) for estimating the *V. vulnificus*/g versus water temperature relationship. A relationship between mean risk versus mean dose was considered more appropriate than a relationship between mean risk and median dose. Both the Exponential and Beta-Poisson dose-response models were considered. When data was grouped or aggregated on a month- and year-specific basis, both the Exponential and Beta-Poisson were found to provide an adequate statistical fit (Table C.2). However, when the data was aggregated on a monthly basis (i.e. risk per month versus dose per month averaged over years), the Beta-Poisson provided a reasonable fit but the Exponential model did not (Table C.3). The MLE fit of the models versus the data are shown in Figures C.1 and C.2.

While neither the Beta-Poisson nor the Exponential model could be rejected when the data was aggregated on a month- and year-specific basis, the resulting predictions based on the maximum likelihood estimate (MLE) of the Beta-Poisson were found to be more consistent with the average monthly or seasonal distribution of illness than the predictions based on the MLE of the Exponential model (Table C.4). The predictions based on the Exponential model were higher than the observed rate of illness in the summer and substantially below the observed rate of illness in the autumn and winter (i.e. predictions were up to ~10-fold lower than observed rates). Consequently, the Beta-Poisson model was considered a more appropriate model for risk characterization.

The sensitivity of the Beta-Poisson model fit to the uncertainty of the *V. vulnificus*/g versus water temperature relationship is shown in Figure C.3. Although the dose-response is shifted depending on the dataset used to estimate the *V. vulnificus*/g versus water temperature relationship, the shape of the relationship is relatively unchanged. Hence, each of these alternative dose-responses predicts seasonal distribution of risk per serving when combined with exposure estimates derived from the respective *V. vulnificus*/g versus water temperature estimates (see Tables D.2 to D.4 in Appendix D).

As indicated above, effects of aggregation bias in the interpretation and analysis of aggregate-level or "grouped" data may preclude using the estimated relationship as pertaining to individual-level risk versus individual-level dose. Consequently, a simulation was conducted to investigate whether or not the estimated relationship for mean risk versus mean dose could be assumed to apply as a relationship between individual-level risk versus individual-level dose (see text box attachment for detail on the simulation). For the fit of the Beta-Poisson model it was determined that (as a consequence of aggregation bias) the obtained relationship of mean risk versus mean dose could not be assumed to apply on the

**Table C.1** Reported cases of oyster-related *V. vulnificus* septicaemia in the USA by month and year.

| Month and year | No. of cases | Annual total | Month and year | No. of cases | Annual total |
|---|---|---|---|---|---|
| Jan-95 | 0 | | Aug-98 | 4 | |
| Feb-95 | 0 | | Sep-98 | 3 | |
| Mar-95 | 0 | | Oct-98 | 4 | |
| Apr-95 | 3 | | Nov-98 | 11 | |
| May-95 | 9 | | Dec-98 | 2 | 40 |
| Jun-95 | 2 | | Jan-99 | 0 | |
| Jul-95 | 2 | | Feb-99 | 1 | |
| Aug-95 | 5 | | Mar-99 | 1 | |
| Sep-95 | 4 | | Apr-99 | 4 | |
| Oct-95 | 5 | | May-99 | 3 | |
| Nov-95 | 2 | | Jun-99 | 3 | |
| Dec-95 | 0 | 32 | Jul-99 | 5 | |
| Jan-96 | 0 | | Aug-99 | 5 | |
| Feb-96 | 0 | | Sep-99 | 8 | |
| Mar-96 | 0 | | Oct-99 | 3 | |
| Apr-96 | 0 | | Nov-99 | 0 | |
| May-96 | 4 | | Dec-99 | 1 | 34 |
| Jun-96 | 4 | | Jan-00 | 0 | |
| Jul-96 | 2 | | Feb-00 | 0 | |
| Aug-96 | 9 | | Mar-00 | 0 | |
| Sep-96 | 4 | | Apr-00 | 0 | |
| Oct-96 | 5 | | May-00 | 4 | |
| Nov-96 | 3 | | Jun-00 | 6 | |
| Dec-96 | 1 | 32 | Jul-00 | 4 | |
| Jan-97 | 1 | | Aug-00 | 5 | |
| Feb-97 | 0 | | Sep-00 | 5 | |
| Mar-97 | 0 | | Oct-00 | 6 | |
| Apr-97 | 0 | | Nov-00 | 0 | |
| May-97 | 6 | | Dec-00 | 0 | 30 |
| Jun-97 | 1 | | Jan-01 | 0 | |
| Jul-97 | 2 | | Feb-01 | 0 | |
| Aug-97 | 2 | | Mar-01 | 1 | |
| Sep-97 | 4 | | Apr-01 | 3 | |
| Oct-97 | 3 | | May-01 | 1 | |
| Nov-97 | 2 | | Jun-01 | 1 | |
| Dec-97 | 0 | 21 | Jul-01 | 11 | |
| Jan-98 | 0 | | Aug-01 | 6 | |
| Feb-98 | 0 | | Sep-01 | 5 | |
| Mar-98 | 0 | | Oct-01 | 5 | |
| Apr-98 | 3 | | Nov-01 | 1 | |
| May-98 | 5 | | Dec-01 | 1 | 35 |
| Jun-98 | 5 | | | | |
| Jul-98 | 3 | | | | |

SOURCE: M. Glatzer, personal communication, 2001.

individual level without introducing a substantial difference in comparison with utilizing and interpreting the dose-response as estimated (i.e. as a relationship between mean risk versus mean dose). Consequently, for the purpose of risk characterization, the estimated dose-response was interpreted as a relation between mean risk versus mean dose and it was not assumed to apply at the level of individuals.

Uncertainty of the fit of the Beta-Poisson Model was obtained by propagating the uncertainty of the parameter estimates of *V. vulnificus*/g versus water temperature relationship through the dose calculations and refitting the dose-response model to obtain a sequence of corresponding (MLE) parameter fits. A total of 100 uncertainty samples of the parameter values of the *V. vulnificus*/g versus water temperature relationship were used to obtain a corresponding uncertainty sample of 100 for the dose-response parameters of the Beta-Poisson.

**Table C.2** Sensitivity of parameter estimates and goodness-of-fit of Beta-Poisson and exponential dose-response fits versus data used to estimate the *V. vulnificus*/g versus water temperature relationship and month- and year-specific doses.

| | Study data used to estimate *V. vulnificus*/g versus water temperature and month- and year-specific mean doses | | |
|---|---|---|---|
| | Motes[(1)] | Tamplin[(2)] | Pooled |
| **Beta-Poisson:** | | | |
| MLE of $\text{Log}_{10}\ \alpha$ | -5.0321 | -4.985 | -5.0067 |
| MLE of $\text{Log}_{10}\ \beta$ | 5.0398 | 5.601 | 5.3591 |
| Variance of MLE of $\text{Log}_{10}\ \alpha$ | 0.00667 | 0.0076 | 0.00706 |
| Variance of MLE of $\text{Log}_{10}\ \beta$ | 0.0184 | 0.0205 | 0.019 |
| -2 logL | 117.8 | 115 | 117.8 |
| -2 sup logL | 51 | 51 | 51 |
| Deviance of the fit | 66.8 | 64 | 66.8 |
| p-value | 0.89 | 0.93 | 0.89 |
| **Exponential Model:** | | | |
| MLE of $\text{Log}_{10}\ \beta$ | -11.29 | -11.65 | -11.509 |
| Variance of MLE of $\text{Log}_{10}\ \beta$ | 0.103 | 0.0912 | 0.097 |
| -2 logL | 118.6 | 114.8 | 114.1 |
| -2 sup logL | 51 | 51 | 51 |
| Deviance of the fit | 67.6 | 63.8 | 63.1 |
| p-value | 0.89 | 0.94 | 0.95 |

NOTES: Deviance of the fit was calculated based on a Poisson likelihood function with logL the value of the likelihood evaluated at the MLE of the model fit and sup logL calculated as the maximum possible value with mean rate equal to the observed month- and year-specific rates of illness; the Deviance (-2 logL - (-2 sup logL)) is (asymptotically) distributed as a Chi-square with degrees of freedom equal to the number of data points (84) minus the number of parameters in the model (2 for the Beta-Poisson and 1 for the exponential); the p-value of the Deviance of the fit is the probability of obtaining a higher Deviance by chance alone; a p-value of <0.05 indicates a significantly poor fit to the data. DATA SETS: (1) Motes *et al.*, 1998. (2) Tamplin et al., 1994.

**Table C.3** Sensitivity of parameter estimates and goodness-of-fit of Beta-Poisson and Exponential Dose-Response fits versus data used to estimate the *V. vulnificus*/g versus water temperature relationship and month-specific doses.

| | Study data used to estimate *V. vulnificus*/g versus water temperature and to estimate month-specific mean doses | | |
|---|---|---|---|
| | Motes *et al.*[(1)] | Tamplin[(2)] | Pooled data |
| **Beta-Poisson:** | | | |
| MLE of Log10 α | -5.01 | -4.99 | -5.03 |
| MLE of Log10 β | 5.08 | 5.55 | 5.24 |
| Std dev of MLE of Log10 α | 0.0903 | 0.095 | 0.084 |
| Std dev of MLE of Log10 β | 0.258 | 0.27 | 0.25 |
| -2 logL | 27.8 | 27.0 | 25.5 |
| -2 sup logL | 12.4 | 12.4 | 12.4 |
| Deviance of the fit [1] | 15.4 | 14.6 | 13.1 |
| p-value | 0.11 | 0.15 | 0.22 |
| **Exponential Model:** | | | |
| MLE of Log10 β | -11.28 | -11.64 | -11.50 |
| Variance of MLE of Log10 β | 0.193 | 0.166 | 0.185 |
| -2 logL | 52.1 | 45.9 | 47.6 |
| -2 sup logL | 12.4 | 12.4 | 12.4 |
| Deviance of the fit | 39.7 | 33.5 | 35.2 |
| p-value | 0.00004 | 0.0004 | 0.0002 |

NOTES: Deviance of the fit was calculated based on a Poisson likelihood function with logL the value of the likelihood evaluated at the MLE of the model fit and sup logL calculated as the maximum possible value with mean rate equal to the observed month- and year-specific rates of illness; the Deviance (-2 logL - (-2 sup logL)) is (asymptotically) distributed as a Chi-square with degrees of freedom equal to the number of data points (12) minus the number of parameters in the model (2 for the Beta-Poisson and 1 for the exponential); the p-value of the Deviance of the fit is the probability of obtaining a higher Deviance by chance alone; a p-value of <0.05 indicates a significantly poor fit to the data. DATA SETS: (1) Motes *et al.*, 1998. (2) Tamplin et al., 1994.

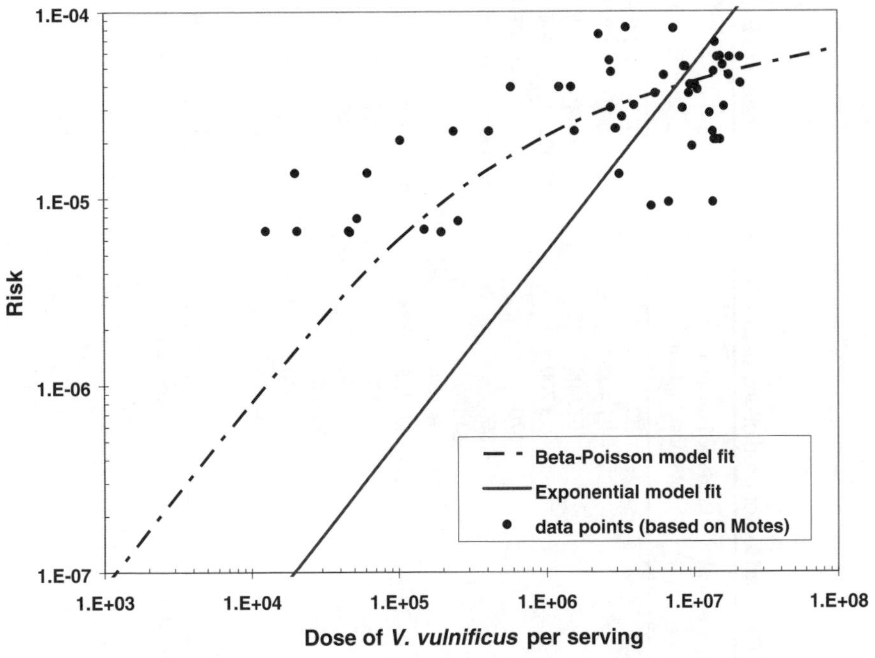


**Figure C.1** Log-Log plot of fit of the Beta-Poisson versus the Exponential model dose-response to mean risk versus estimated mean doses (based on Motes et al. (1998) data; averaged replicates).

**Table C.4** Comparison of predictions of the Beta-Poisson versus the Exponential models.

| Monthly or seasonal grouping | Predicted mean *Vv*/g at consumption | Mean dose | MLE risk prediction of | | Predicted cases based on | | Observed average number of cases |
|---|---|---|---|---|---|---|---|
| | | | Beta-Poisson | Exponential | Beta-Poisson | Exponential | |
| Winter | 80 | 16 000 | 1.27E-06 | 8.21E-08 | 0.52 | 0.03 | 0.57 |
| Spring | 21 400 | 4 280 000 | 3.43E-05 | 2.20E-05 | 11.86 | 7.59 | 9.57 |
| Summer | 57 000 | 11 400 000 | 4.32E-05 | 5.85E-05 | 12.28 | 16.60 | 13.99 |
| Autumn | 3 700 | 740 000 | 1.90E-05 | 3.80E-06 | 8.03 | 1.60 | 7.85 |
| Jan | 70 | 14 000 | 1.12E-06 | 7.18E-08 | 0.14 | 0.01 | 0.14 |
| Feb | 350 | 70 000 | 4.59E-06 | 3.59E-07 | 0.61 | 0.05 | 0.14 |
| Mar | 545 | 109 000 | 6.41E-06 | 5.59E-07 | 0.97 | 0.08 | 0.29 |
| Apr | 3 375 | 675 000 | 1.83E-05 | 3.46E-06 | 2.39 | 0.45 | 1.86 |
| May | 25 125 | 5 025 000 | 3.57E-05 | 2.58E-05 | 3.93 | 2.83 | 4.57 |
| Jun | 57 805 | 11 561 000 | 4.34E-05 | 5.93E-05 | 4.55 | 6.23 | 3.14 |
| Jul | 77 990 | 15 598 000 | 4.61E-05 | 8.00E-05 | 4.47 | 7.76 | 4.14 |
| Aug | 82 680 | 16 536 000 | 4.67E-05 | 8.48E-05 | 4.11 | 7.46 | 5.14 |
| Sep | 45 040 | 9 008 000 | 4.11E-05 | 4.62E-05 | 4.07 | 4.57 | 4.71 |
| Oct | 9 715 | 1 943 000 | 2.72E-05 | 9.96E-06 | 3.46 | 1.27 | 4.43 |
| Nov | 1 285 | 257 000 | 1.12E-05 | 1.32E-06 | 1.64 | 0.19 | 2.71 |
| Dec | 195 | 39 000 | 2.83E-06 | 2.00E-07 | 0.42 | 0.03 | 0.71 |

NOTES: *V. vulnificus*/g versus water temperature relationship estimated based on the Motes et al. (1998) study data (average of replicates considered a single sample).

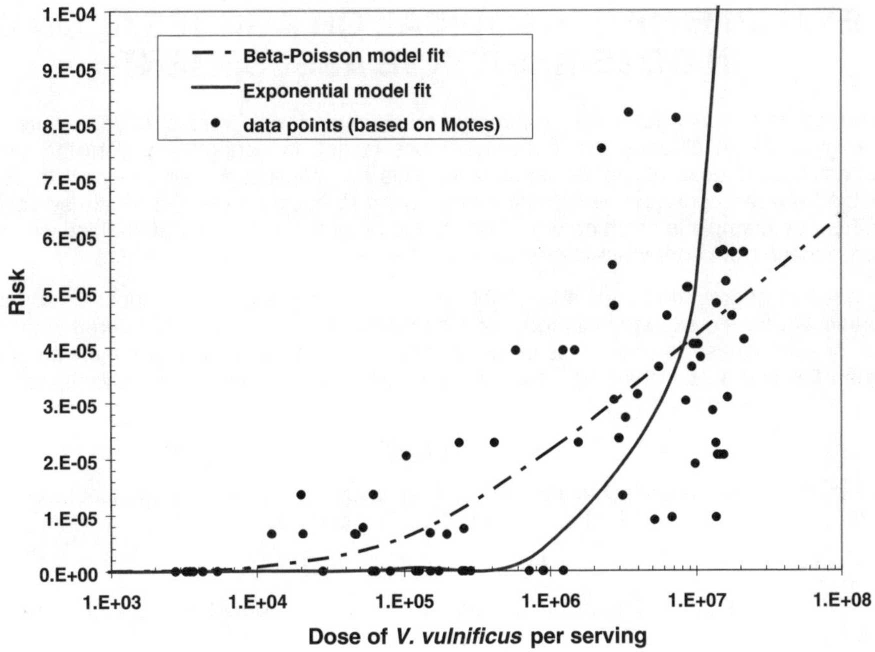


**Figure C.2** Semi-Log plot of fit of the Beta-Poisson versus the Exponential model dose-response to mean risk versus estimated mean doses (based on Motes et al. (1998) data; averaged replicates).

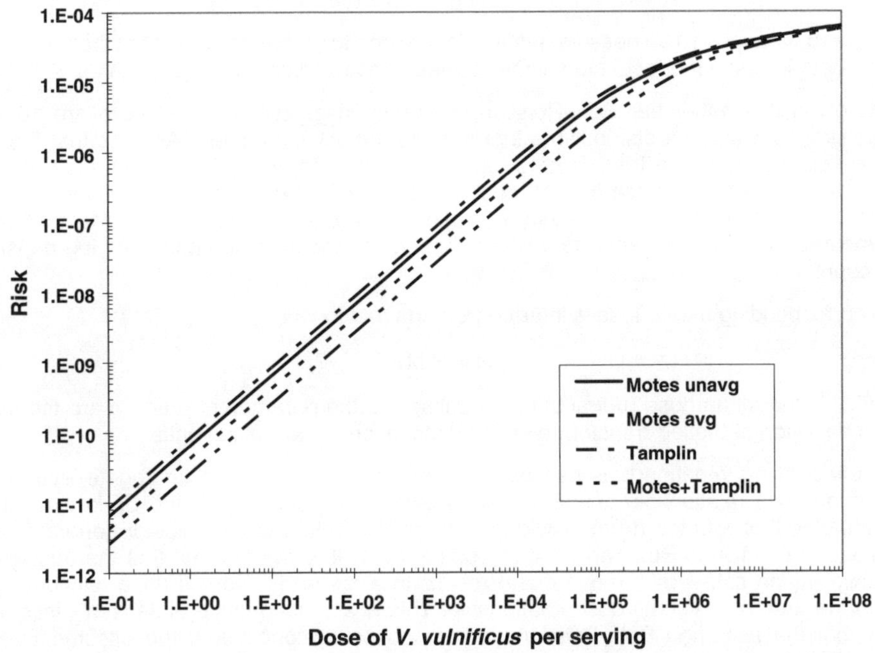


**Figure C.3** Uncertainty of the Beta-Poisson dose-response (mean risk versus mean dose) depending upon the data set used to estimate the *V. vulnificus*/g versus water temperature relationship.

# AN EXAMPLE OF ECOLOGICAL OR AGGREGATION BIAS IN DOSE-RESPONSE ASSESSMENT

A relationship between aggregate (summary) measures of risk versus dose across a set of exposure groups with differing distributions of dose is not, in general, equal to the relationship between risk versus dose at the individual level. This has implications with respect to how well a relationship between aggregate-level data can be used to estimate the individual risk versus dose relationship. An example is given here to illustrate the potential magnitude of the bias when such an inference is made from aggregate-level data.

The issue of aggregation bias is negligible when the dose-response is linear or approximately so. In particular, for the exponential model or 1-hit model, which may be considered appropriate for microbial dose-response for low levels of exposure or risk, the risk is approximately proportional to dose when the risk is less than $10^{-3}$. Hence, for doses corresponding to risks less than $10^{-3}$, the dose-response would be well approximated by

$$P(d) = \beta^{*}d$$

Any aggregate-level relationship that derives from such a linear underlying model would itself be unbiased with respect to the individual-level relationship because

$$E[P(D_i)] = E[\beta^{*}D_i] = \beta^{*}E[D_i]$$

for any sequence of dose distribution $D_i$ generating the aggregate-level relationship of $E[P(D_i)]$ versus $E[D_i]$.

The situation is different if the dose-response is non-linear. Assume that the true individual-level risk of infection at a given dose $d$ is binomially distributed with mean risk $P(d)$ given by the following function (approximate Beta-Poisson):

$$P(d) = 1 - (1+d/\beta)^{-\alpha}$$

with $\alpha = 1\times10^{-6}$ and $\beta = 10^{5}$. These values are (approximately) that of the best estimates obtained in fitting the Beta-Poisson model to the estimated mean dose versus mean risk data for *V. vulnificus*.

Now, given this non-linear Beta-Poisson dose-response, assume that there are 10 separate exposure groups with dose distributions that are lognormally distributed. Assume that the mean of the dose distributions range from 1 to 10 $\log_{10}$ by increments of 1 (i.e. 10, 100, etc.) and that the standard deviation of $\log_{10}$ dose is fixed at 1.4 across all 10 exposure groups. These distributions represent the variation of density of colony forming units (cfu) per exposure and "actual" individual level exposure would be assumed to follow a Poisson distribution about the varying density of cfu per exposure.

The corresponding mean dose is inferred from the relationship:

$$E[D] = \exp(\mu + \sigma^{2}/2)$$

where $E[D]$ is the mean dose (untransformed units) and the parameters $\mu$ and $\sigma$ are the mean and standard deviation of the log-transformed dose distribution in natural log units.

The effect of aggregation bias can be illustrated by computing the aggregate-level mean risk versus mean dose relationship across these 10 exposure groups by Monte Carlo simulation, and then comparing that with the (true) individual-level relationship that underlies or generates it. These calculations are shown in Box Table 1 and Box Figure 1. It is evident that that the aggregate-level relationship (mean risk versus mean dose) results in a mean risk versus dose relationship that is less than the "true" risk versus dose relationship. This is a consequence of Jensen's inequality and the fact that the assumed Beta-Poisson dose-response is concave. If the assumed true dose-response were convex, then the aggregate-level risk versus dose relationship would be greater than the true risk versus dose relationship.

**Box Table 1**. Calculation of the aggregate-level mean risk versus mean dose relationship across the 10 exposure groups by Monte Carlo simulation.

| Individual-level $Log_{10}$ dose | Individual-level dose | Individual-level risk | Aggregate-level mean dose | Simulated(1) mean risk |
|---|---|---|---|---|
| 1 | $10^1$ | 1.00E-10 | $3.3 \times 10^2$ | 9.01E-11 |
| 2 | $10^2$ | 1.00E-09 | $3.3 \times 10^3$ | 7.61E-10 |
| 3 | $10^3$ | 9.95E-09 | $3.3 \times 10^4$ | 5.40E-09 |
| 4 | $10^4$ | 9.53E-08 | $3.3 \times 10^5$ | 3.07E-08 |
| 5 | $10^5$ | 6.93E-07 | $3.3 \times 10^6$ | 1.36E-07 |
| 6 | $10^6$ | 2.40E-06 | $3.3 \times 10^7$ | 4.57E-07 |
| 7 | $10^7$ | 4.62E-06 | $3.3 \times 10^8$ | 1.20E-06 |
| 8 | $10^8$ | 6.91E-06 | $3.3 \times 10^9$ | 2.48E-06 |
| 9 | $10^9$ | 9.21E-06 | $3.3 \times 10^{10}$ | 4.28E-06 |
| 10 | $10^{10}$ | 1.15E-05 | $3.3 \times 10^{11}$ | 6.38E-06 |

NOTE: (1) Based on simple random sample of size $n = 10^8$, giving a relative error of <1% for the simulated mean dose versus true mean dose for each of the 10 dose groups.

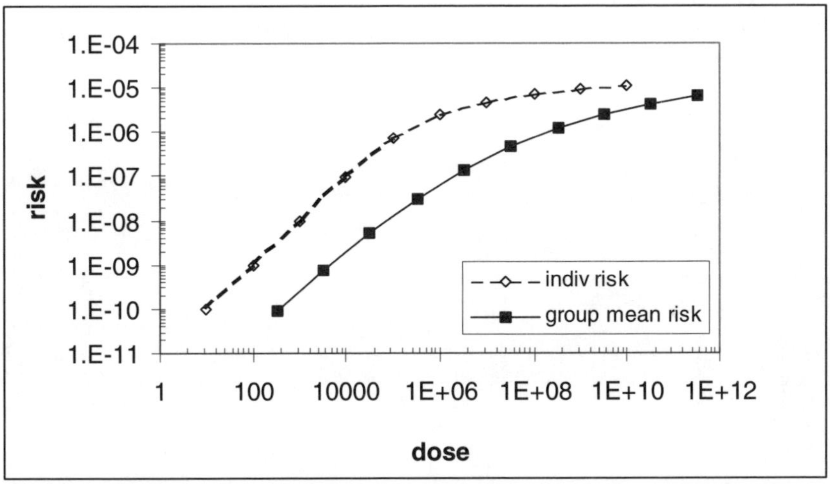


**Box Figure 1.** Comparison of the aggregate-level relationship (mean risk versus mean dose) with the "true" risk versus dose relationship.

## Further reading

Crump, K.S. 1998. On summarizing group exposures in risk assessment: is an arithmetic mean or a geometric mean more appropriate? *Risk Analysis*, **18**(3): 293–329.

Haas, C.N. 1996. How to average microbial densities to characterize risk. *Water Research*, **30**(4): 1036–1038

# REFERENCES

Crump, K.S. 1998. On summarizing group exposures in risk assessment: is an arithmetic mean or a geometric mean more appropriate? *Risk Analysis*, **18**(3): 293–297.

Greenland, S. & Morgenstern, H. 1989. Ecological bias, confounding, and effect modification. *International Journal of Epidemiology*, **18**(1): 269–274.

Motes, M.L., DePaola, A., Cook, D.W., Veazey, J.E., Hunsucker, J.C., Garthright, W.E., Blodgett, R.J. & Chirtel, S.J. 1998. Influence of water temperature and salinity on *Vibrio vulnificus* in northern Gulf and Atlantic Coast oysters (*Crassostrea virginica*). *Applied and Environmental Microbiology,* **64**: 1459–1465.

Piantadosi, S., Byar, D. & Green, S. 1988. The ecological fallacy. *American Journal of Epidemiology*, **127**(6): 893–904.

Richardson, S., Stucker, I. & Hemon, D. 1987. Comparison of relative risks obtained in ecological and individual studies: some methodological considerations. *International Journal of Epidemiology*, **16**(1): 111–120.

Tamplin, M.L. 1994. The seasonal occurrence of *Vibrio vulnificus* in shellfish, seawater, and sediment in United States coastal waters. Final report to Salstonstall-Kennedy Grant Program, US Department of Commerce.

# COMPARATIVE RESULTS OF ASSESSMENT BASED ON ALTERNATIVE DATA SETS FOR RELATIONSHIP BETWEEN *V. VULNIFICUS* PER GRAM AND WATER TEMPERATURE AT HARVEST

Given uncertainty as to the appropriate data set for estimation of the *V. vulnificus/g* versus water temperature relationship, the sensitivity of the risk assessment to this uncertainty was evaluated by performing replicate analyses with different estimates of this relationship. This relationship underlies both the risk characterization and the dose-response assessment.

The resulting differences in the estimated dose-response relationship are shown in Appendix C. Here, the effect of using different data sets on the exposure and risk estimates obtained for risk characterization is summarized. These estimates are compared with retail study data on levels of *V. vulnificus* at (or close to) the point of consumption. Additionally the sensitivity of low-dose risk predictions to alternative estimates of the *V. vulnificus/g* versus water temperature relationship are given.

Seasonal dose and risk predictions are given in Tables D.1 through D.4 for each of four alternative approaches for estimating the *V. vulnificus/g* versus water temperature relationship. The alternatives considered were: (1) Motes et al. (1998) data with replicate samples considered distinct; (2) Motes et al. data with replicate data considered non-distinct and therefore averaged; (3) Tamplin data (Tamplin et al., 1982); and (4) pooling the Motes et al. (unaveraged replicate data) with the Tamplin data set.

With respect to the numbers presented in Tables D.1 through D.4, it is immediately evident that the number of cases, both per annum and seasonally, are not appreciably different. This is to be expected since for each of the four alternative approaches the estimated *V. vulnificus/g* versus water temperature relationship underlies the dose-response assessment as well as the risk characterization. Consequently, while there are obvious differences in the predicted seasonal mean *V. vulnificus*/g (e.g. much higher when based on Tamplin data compared with that obtained when based on Motes et al. data), the same level of risk is effectively attributed to these different dose levels.

Validation of the model-predicted seasonal exposure estimates is provided by comparison with independent data on the levels of *V. vulnificus*/g in retail oysters. These data were not used for estimation of model parameters and therefore provide a check of the predictions of the model based on alternative estimates of the *V. vulnificus/g* versus water temperature relationship at the time of harvest. A graphical comparison is shown in Figures D.1 to D.4. In Figures D.1 to D.3, the predicted versus observed mean $\log_{10}$ *V. vulnificus*/g are shown, along with 90% uncertainty intervals for the mean. For the retail data, the 95% confidence interval for the mean is shown. From these graphs it is evident that there is little appreciable difference in the predicted mean $\log_{10}$ *V. vulnificus*/g levels in the spring or summer based on Motes et al. compared with Tamplin. The predictions based on the combination of these data is most similar to the results based on Motes et al. data alone; a consequence of the fact that there are twice as many observations in this data set compared with the Tamplin set. With respect to the winter and autumn, the predictions based on the Tamplin data are noticeably lower than those based on the Motes et al. data set. However, the differences are not substantial.

More pronounced differences in predictions of exposure based on Motes et al. versus Tamplin data sets are shown in Figure D.4. Here the effect of differences in estimates of population variation of $\log_{10}$ *V. vulnificus*/g levels is evident. Predicted mean *V. vulnificus*/g is a function of both the mean and variation of $\log_{10}$ *V. vulnificus*/g (i.e. *V. vulnificus*/g has a positively skewed distribution). In comparing model-predicted mean *V. vulnificus*/g with retail-data-based estimates, it should be noted that the retail estimates are likely to be biased high. This is because the estimates based on the retail data have not been adjusted for method error, which has generally been shown to be symmetric on the log scale. The retail data was not adjusted for method error here because the magnitude of the method error is not known exactly, as a consequence of interference from other microbial species in the confirmation step of the MPN procedure.

While the magnitude to which estimates of mean *V. vulnificus*/g are biased high based on the retail data is somewhat problematic, there are evident differences between the comparative predictions based on the Motes et al. data compared with that of the Tamplin data. In particular, for the summer season the mean *V. vulnificus*/g predicted based on the Tamplin data set is 132 000/g, which is 2-fold higher than prediction based on the Motes et al. data. The mean based on the retail data, while still likely to be biased high, is much more consistent with the predictions based on the Motes et al. data. The prediction of mean levels based on 1998/1999 autumn- and winter-specific water temperatures (Figure D.4) are considerably higher than that indicated by the retail data, particularly for the winter season.

The implications of the uncertainty (as to appropriate data for estimation of the *V. vulnificus*/g versus water temperature relationship) on low-dose risk predictions is shown in Table D.5. While the differences between considering replicate samples to be independent collections versus not independent in analysis of the Motes et al. data appear to be minor; there are more substantial differences in predictions of risk and illness burden at target levels of 3/g, 30/g and 300/g when the assessment is based on Motes et al. data compared with that obtained when it is based on the Tamplin data. At a standard of 3/g, the projected illness burden is 0.1 versus 0.02 cases per year, based on the Motes et al. data and Tamplin data sets, respectively.

The apparent differences between the Motes et al. and Tamplin data sets are confirmed by a statistical analysis of the goodness-of-fit of the assumed regression model to the pooled data in comparison with the fit of the model to each dataset separately. The likelihood ratio statistic is an appropriate goodness-of-fit measure for this comparison. The pooling of data is reasonable if, in the context of the assumed model, there are no appreciable or significant differences between the fit of the model to one data set compared with the other. Specifically, with respect to the issue of pooling Tamplin and the Motes et al. data sets to estimate the $\log_{10}$ *V. vulnificus*/g versus water temperature relationship, the likelihood ratio statistic is of the form:

$$LR = \frac{\hat{L}_{pooled}}{\hat{L}_{Motes}\hat{L}_{Tamplin}}$$

or

$$-2\ln(LR) = -2\left(\ln(\hat{L}_{pooled}) - (\ln(\hat{L}_{Motes}) + \ln(\hat{L}_{Tamplin}))\right)$$

where

$\hat{L}_{pooled}$ is the maximized value of the likelihood of the pooled data

$\hat{L}_{Motes}$ is the maximized value of the likelihood of the Motes data (separately)

$\hat{L}_{Tamplin}$ is the maximized value of the likelihood of the Tamplin data (separately)

The log of the likelihood ratio statistic has a chi - square distribution :

$$-2\ln(LR) \sim \chi_{p-q}$$

where

p = number of parameters for fits to Motes and Tamplin separately

q = number of parameters for fit of Motes and Tamplin pooled together

Fitting of a quadratic temperature effect regression model to $\log_{10}$ *V. vulnificus*/g by the censored regression method resulted in maximized log likelihoods of -295.2, -375.9 and -714.9 for the Tamplin data alone, Motes et al. (unaveraged replicates) data alone and for the pooled data sets, respectively. Thus, from the equation above, the likelihood ratio statistic has the value 87.6. With respect to the pooled data set, a model with 4 parameters is being fitted (intercept, linear and quadratic terms in temperature and a residual variance parameter). When the data sets are fitted separately the total number of parameters is 8. Thus, under the null hypothesis that the two data sets are consistent with the same parameter values, the likelihood ratio statistic is distributed as a chi-square with 4 degrees of freedom. The $95^{th}$ percentile of the Chi-square distribution with 4 degrees of freedom is 9.48. Hence, given that the observed chi-square (87.6) is greater than the $95^{th}$ percentile, the hypothesis that the two data sets are consistent with the same set of parameter values can be rejected at the 95% confidence level.

Specifically, the hypothesis tested by the likelihood ratio statistic is:

$$H_o : \underline{\theta}_{Motes} = \underline{\theta}_{Tamplin} \quad versus \quad H_A : \underline{\theta}_{Motes} \neq \underline{\theta}_{Tamplin}$$

where

$\underline{\theta} = (\alpha, \beta, \gamma, \sigma)$, the parameter vector of the quadratic regression model

The likelihood ratio statistic is not a specific test as to which component of the population parameter vector is appreciably different for one data set versus another. However, inspection of the maximum likelihood parameter estimates obtained (Appendix B) indicates that there is little difference between the α, β and γ parameters and a large difference with respect to the estimate of σ. Based on the likelihood ratio test, this difference is significant enough to advise against pooling of the data.

**Table D.1** Summary (median and 90% intervals of uncertainty distribution) of model predictions for mean exposure and risk assuming estimate of *V. vulnificus*/g versus water temperature based on the Motes et al. study (unaveraged replicates considered independent samples).

| Season | $Log_{10}$ *V. vulnificus*/g at harvest | *V. vulnificus*/g at harvest | $Log_{10}$ *V. vulnificus*/g at consumption | *V. vulnificus*/g at consumption | Risk per serving | Predicted number of cases(2) |
|---|---|---|---|---|---|---|
| Winter (Jan – Mar) | 0.38 | 50 | 0.22 | 100 | $1.31\times10^{-6}$ | 0.5 (0.1, 2.5) |
| | (-0.44, 0.91) | (10, 140) | (-0.68, 0.83) | (30, 600) | $(2.51\times10^{-7}, 5.97\times10^{-6})$ | |
| Spring (Apr – Jun) | 2.74 | 3 700 | 3.29 | 25 900 | $3.32\times10^{-5}$ | 11.5 (9.8, 14.0) |
| | (2.40, 2.97) | (2 500, 5 700) | (2.77, 3.64) | (17 600, 39 800) | $(2.84\times10^{-5}, 4.08\times10^{-5})$ | |
| Summer (Jul – Sept) | 3.27 | 7 900 | 4.14 | 65 300 | $4.28\times10^{-5}$ | 12.1 (10.4, 13.8) |
| | (3.18, 3.35) | (6 100, 10 800) | (4.03, 4.24) | (54 000, 78 600) | $(3.67\times10^{-5}, 4.87\times10^{-5})$ | |
| Autumn (Oct – Dec) | 1.33 | 720 | 1.39 | 4 800 | $1.86\times10^{-5}$ | 7.8 (4.7, 11.8) |
| | (0.24, 2.02) | (380, 1 400) | (0.14, 2.28) | (2 100, 12 000) | $(1.12\times10^{-5}, 2.80\times10^{-5})$ | |
| Autumn 1998(1) | 2.52 | 2 500 | 2.98 | 19 200 | $3.11\times10^{-5}$ | 13.1 (11.7, 15.0) |
| | (2.42, 2.62) | (1 900, 3 500) | (2.86, 3.08) | (16 300, 22 800) | $(2.77\times10^{-5}, 3.55\times10^{-5})$ | |
| Winter 1999(1) | 1.06 | 160 | 1.03 | 500 | $4.84\times10^{-6}$ | 2.0 (1.1, 3.1) |
| | (0.91, 1.19) | (110, 220) | (0.88, 1.16) | (330, 710) | $(2.73\times10^{-6}, 7.53\times10^{-6})$ | |

NOTES: (1) Predictions based on water temperature distributions for Weeks Bay, Alabama, USA, in 1998 and 1999. (2) Based on number of servings (from Table 13 in Technical Report).

**Table D.2** Summary (median and 90% intervals of uncertainty distribution) of model predictions for mean exposure and risk assuming estimate of *V. vulnificus*/g versus water temperature based on the Motes et al. study (average of replicates considered a single sample).

| Month | $Log_{10}$ *V. vulnificus*/g at harvest | *V. vulnificus*/g at harvest | $Log_{10}$ *V. vulnificus*/g at consumption | *V. vulnificus*/g at consumption | Risk per serving | Predicted number of cases(2) |
|---|---|---|---|---|---|---|
| Winter | 0.47 | 40 | 0.30 | 80 | $1.26\times10^{-6}$ | 0.5 |
| (Jan–Mar) | (-0.39, 1.04) | (10, 140) | (-0.60, 1.01) | (20, 610) | $(2.92\times10^{-7}, 6.71\times10^{-6})$ | (0.1, 2.8) |
| Spring | 2.75 | 2,600 | 3.28 | 21,400 | $3.37\times10^{-5}$ | 11.7 |
| (Apr–Jun) | (2.39, 2.97) | (1 600, 3 900) | (2.80, 3.61) | (12 700, 33 500) | $(2.83\times10^{-5}, 4.05\times10^{-5})$ | (9.8, 14.0) |
| Summer | 3.27 | 5 600 | 4.15 | 57 000 | $4.28\times10^{-5}$ | 12.2 |
| (Jul–Sept) | (3.09, 3.41) | (3 200, 7 800) | (3.95, 4.29) | (37 900, 70 500) | $(3.69\times10^{-5}, 4.97\times10^{-5})$ | (10.5, 14.1) |
| Autumn | 1.39 | 500 | 1.45 | 3,700 | $1.92\times10^{-5}$ | 8.0 |
| (Oct–Dec) | (0.33, 2.06) | (220, 1 100) | (0.26, 2.32) | (1 500, 11 700) | $(1.30\times10^{-5}, 2.82\times10^{-5})$ | (5.5, 11.9) |
| Autumn 1998(1) | 2.54 | 1 700 | 2.99 | 16 100 | $3.11\times10^{-5}$ | 13.1 |
| | (2.41, 2.68) | (1 100, 2 400) | (2.86, 3.12) | (11 800, 19 800) | $(2.78\times10^{-5}, 3.57\times10^{-5})$ | (11.7, 15.0) |
| Winter 1999(1) | 1.11 | 110 | 1.08 | 390 | $4.87\times10^{-6}$ | 2.0 |
| | (0.90, 1.31) | (80, 170) | (0.87, 1.28) | (240, 590) | $(2.93\times10^{-6}, 7.74\times10^{-6})$ | (1.2, 3.2) |

NOTES: (1) Predictions based on water temperature distributions for Weeks Bay, Alabama, USA, in 1998 and 1999. (2) Based on number of servings (from Table 13 in Technical Report).

**Table D.3** Summary (median and 90% intervals of uncertainty distribution) of model predictions for mean exposure and risk assuming estimate of *V. vulnificus*/g versus water temperature based on the Tamplin study.

| Month | $Log_{10}$ *V. vulnificus*/g at harvest | *V. vulnificus*/g at harvest | $Log_{10}$ *V. vulnificus*/g at consumption | *V. vulnificus*/g at consumption | Risk per serving | Predicted number of cases[(2)] |
|---|---|---|---|---|---|---|
| Winter | -0.90 | 110 | -1.05 | 240 | $1.25\times10^{-6}$ | 0.5 |
| (Jan – Mar) | (-2.13, 0.02) | (20, 960) | (-2.37, -0.04) | (30, 1 800) | ($1.79\times10^{-7}$, $6.31\times10^{-6}$) | (0.07, 2.6) |
| Spring | 2.42 | 26,800 | 2.89 | 55 300 | $3.34\times10^{-5}$ | 11.6 |
| (Apr – Jun) | (1.79, 3.00) | (7,600, 55,500) | (2.22, 3.56) | (21 800, 92 100) | ($2.85\times10^{-5}$, $4.09\times10^{-5}$) | (9.9, 14.2) |
| Summer | 3.38 | 66,100 | 4.15 | 131 800 | $4.30\ 10^{-5}$ | 12.2 |
| (Jul – Sept) | (2.67, 3.96) | (16,400, 131,900) | (3.49, 4.60) | (63 100, 203 000) | ($3.66\times10^{-5}$, $4.89\times10^{-5}$) | (10.4, 13.9) |
| Autumn | 0.43 | 4,100 | 0.46 | 9 200 | $1.77\ 10^{-5}$ | 7.5 |
| (Oct – Dec) | (-1.01, 1.39) | (1 000, 12,500) | (-1.07, 1.65) | (3 300, 25 600) | ($1.20\times10^{-5}$, $2.59\times10^{-5}$) | (5.1, 11.0) |
| Autumn 1998[(1)] | 2.06 | 16,100 | 2.49 | 36 600 | $2.98\ 10^{-5}$ | 12.6 |
| | (1.57, 2.53) | (5,200, 34 000) | (2.01, 2.92) | (16 600, 59 800) | ($2.68\times10^{-5}$, $3.44\times10^{-5}$) | (11.3, 14.5) |
| Winter 1999[(1)] | -0.03 | 550 | -0.05 | 1,100 | $4.61\ 10^{-6}$ | 1.9 |
| | (-0.43, 0.37) | (150, 1,400) | (-0.46, 0.35) | (400, 2 200) | ($2.18\times10^{-6}$, $7.94\times10^{-6}$) | (0.9, 3.3) |

NOTES: (1) Predictions based on water temperature distributions for Weeks Bay, Alabama, USA, in 1998 and 1999. (2) Based on number of servings (from Table 13 in Technical Report).

**Table D.4** Summary (median and 90% intervals of uncertainty distribution) of model predictions for mean exposure and risk assuming estimate of *V. vulnificus*/g versus water temperature based on pooled Motes et al. and Tamplin study data.

| Month | $Log_{10}$ *V. vulnificus*/g at harvest | *V. vulnificus*/g at harvest | $Log_{10}$ *V. vulnificus*/g at consumption | *V. vulnificus*/g at consumption | Risk per serving | Predicted number of cases[(2)] |
|---|---|---|---|---|---|---|
| Winter | -0.17 | 70 | -0.32 | 140 | $1.22\times10^{-6}$ | 0.5 |
| (Jan–Mar) | (-1.05, 0.49) | (20, 310) | (-1.26, 0.44) | (20, 1 000) | ($2.56\times10^{-7}$, $6.65\times10^{-6}$) | (0.1, 2.7) |
| Spring | 2.59 | 9,300 | 3.13 | 36 600 | $3.34\times10^{-5}$ | 11.6 |
| (Apr–Jun) | (2.15, 2.84) | (5 600, 13 700) | (2.53, 3.50) | (24 100, 55 800) | ($2.85\times10^{-5}$, $4.10\times10^{-5}$) | (9.9, 14.2) |
| Summer | 3.30 | 22 700 | 4.13 | 93 400 | $4.31\times10^{-5}$ | 12.2 |
| (Jul–Sept) | (3.16, 3.41) | (15 200, 29 300) | (3.97, 4.25) | (72 900, 107 000) | ($3.66\times10^{-5}$, $4.89\times10^{-5}$) | (10.4, 13.9) |
| Autumn | 0.92 | 1 500 | 0.99 | 6 100 | $1.85\times10^{-5}$ | 7.8 |
| (Oct–Dec) | (-0.19, 1.71) | (700, 4 000) | (-0.23, 1.96) | (2 700, 16 500) | ($1.28\times10^{-5}$, $2.66\times10^{-5}$) | (5.4, 11.2) |
| Autumn 1998[(1)] | 2.32 | 5 600 | 2.76 | 25 400 | $3.02\times10^{-5}$ | 12.7 |
| | (2.24, 2.42) | (4 100, 7 700) | (2.68, 2.87) | (21 100, 28 800) | ($2.72\times10^{-5}$, $3.48\times10^{-5}$) | (11.5, 14.7) |
| Winter 1999[(1)] | 0.62 | 240 | 0.59 | 670 | $4.65\times10^{-6}$ | 1.9 |
| | (0.46, 0.77) | (150, 380) | (0.43, 0.74) | (420, 1 000) | ($2.45\times10^{-6}$, $7.57\times10^{-6}$) | (1.0, 3.1) |

NOTES: (1) Predictions based on water temperature distributions for Weeks Bay, Alabama, USA, in 1998 and 1999. (2) Based on number of servings (from Table 13 in Technical Report).

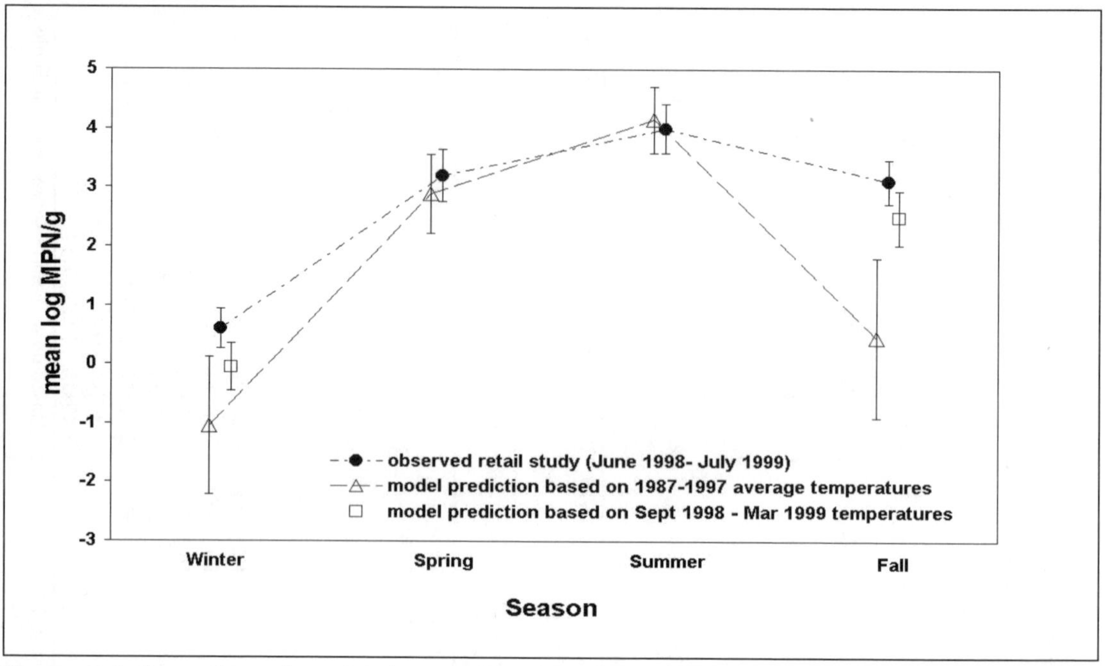


**Figure D.1** Comparison of predicted mean $\log_{10}$ *V. vulnificus*/g based on Motes et al. (unaveraged replicates) data versus independent estimate of $\log_{10}$ *V. vulnificus*/g based on retail data (Cook et al., 2002).

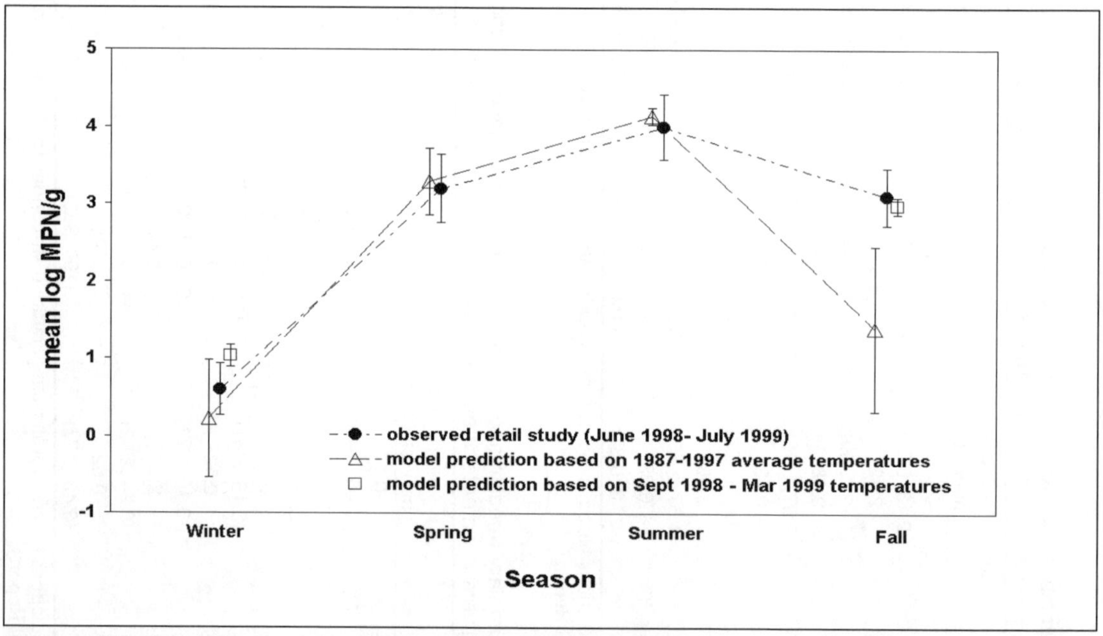


**Figure D.2** Comparison of predicted mean $\log_{10}$ *V. vulnificus*/g based on Tamplin data with independent estimate of $\log_{10}$ *V. vulnificus*/g based on retail data (Cook et al., 2002).

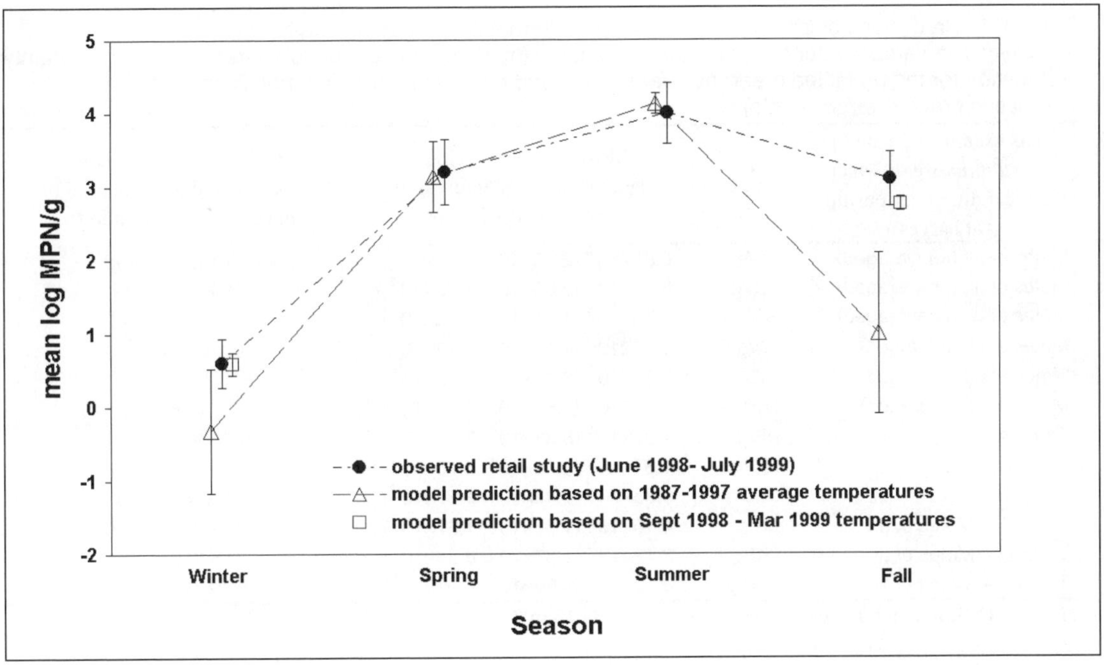


**Figure D.3** Comparison of predicted mean $\log_{10}$ *V. vulnificus*/g based on combined Motes et al. (unaveraged replicates) and Tamplin data versus independent estimate of $\log_{10}$ *V. vulnificus*/g based on retail data (Cook et al., 2002).

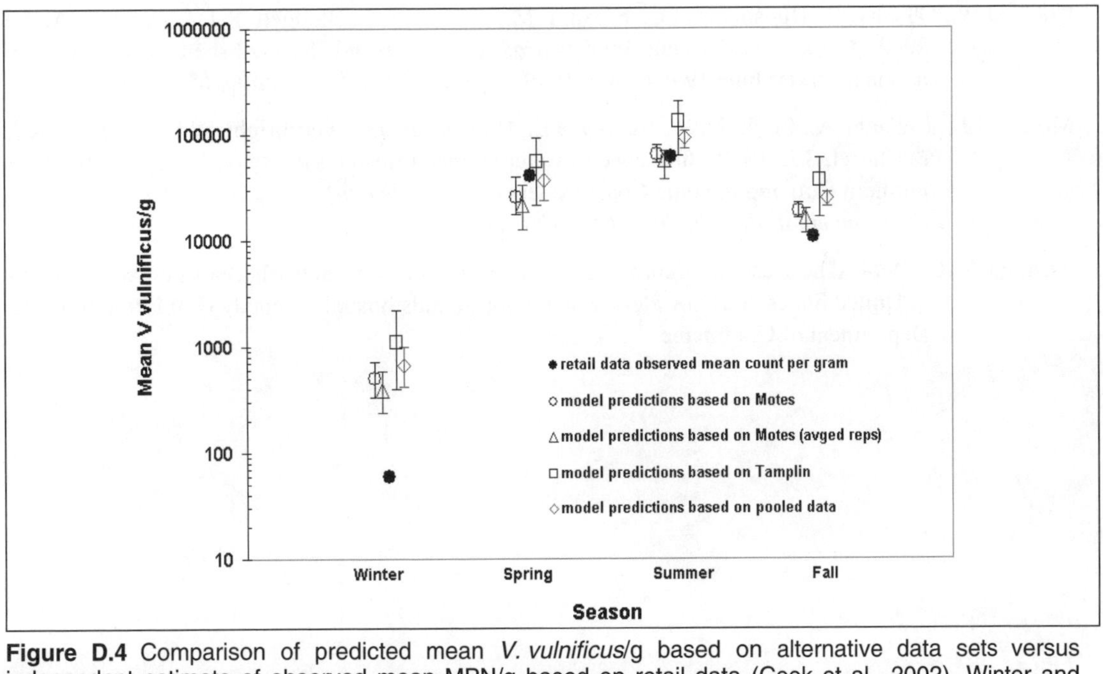


**Figure D.4** Comparison of predicted mean *V. vulnificus*/g based on alternative data sets versus independent estimate of observed mean MPN/g based on retail data (Cook et al., 2002). Winter and autumn model predictions are based on 1998/99-specific water temperatures.

**Table D.5** Predictions of low-dose risk based on alternative data sets used to estimate the *V. vulnificus*/g versus water temperature relationship (median and central 90% interval of the uncertainty distribution for the predicted mean risk per serving and mean annual number of illnesses for three alternative process target levels).

| Data used to estimate the *V. vulnificus*/g vs water temperature relationship (at harvest) | Target | Mean risk per serving (median and 90% interval of uncertainty distribution) | Annual number of cases (median and 90% interval of uncertainty distribution)(1) |
|---|---|---|---|
| Motes et al. (unaveraged) | 3/g | $6.83\times10^{-8}$ ($2.73\times10^{-8}$, $2.05\times10^{-7}$) | 0.1 (0.04, 0.3) |
| Motes et al. (unaveraged) | 30/g | $5.46\times10^{-7}$ ($2.05\times10^{-7}$, $1.43\times10^{-6}$) | 0.8 (0.3, 2.1) |
| Motes et al. (unaveraged) | 300/g | $3.76\times10^{-6}$ ($1.71\times10^{-6}$, $8.33\times10^{-6}$) | 5.5 (2.5, 12.2) |
| Motes et al. (averaged) | 3/g | $1.09\times10^{-7}$ ($4.10\times10^{-8}$, $2.73\times10^{-7}$) | 0.16 (0.06, 0.4) |
| Motes et al. (averaged) | 30/g | $8.20\times10^{-7}$ ($3.42\times10^{-7}$, $2.12\times10^{-6}$) | 1.2 (0.5, 3.1) |
| Motes et al. (averaged) | 300/g | $5.26\times10^{-6}$ ($2.60\times10^{-6}$, $1.05\times10^{-6}$) | 7.7 (3.8, 15.3) |
| Tamplin | 3/g | $1.37\times10^{-8}$ ($6.83\times10^{-9}$, $7.51\times10^{-8}$) | 0.02 (0.01, 0.11) |
| Tamplin | 30/g | $1.37\times10^{-7}$ ($4.78\times10^{-8}$, $4.78\times10^{-7}$) | 0.2 (0.07, 0.7) |
| Tamplin | 300/g | $8.88\times10^{-7}$ ($3.42\times10^{-7}$, $2.87\times10^{-6}$) | 1.3 (0.5, 4.2) |
| Tamplin + Motes et al. | 3/g | $4.10\times10^{-8}$ ($1.37\times10^{-8}$, $1.37\times10^{-7}$) | 0.06 (0.02, 0.2) |
| Tamplin + Motes et al. | 30/g | $3.42\times10^{-7}$ ($1.37\times10^{-7}$, $8.54\times10^{-7}$) | 0.5 (0.2, 1.25) |
| Tamplin + Motes et al. | 300/g | $2.12\times10^{-6}$ ($9.56\times10^{-7}$, $4.99\times10^{-6}$) | 3.1 (1.4, 7.3) |

NOTES: (1) Based on number of servings (from Table 13 in Technical Report).

# REFERENCES

Cook, D.W., O'Leary, P., Hunsucker, J.C., Sloan, E.M., Bowers, J.C., Blodgett, R.J. & DePaola, A. 2002. *Vibrio vulnificus* and *Vibrio parahaemolyticus* in U.S. retail shell oysters: A national survey June 1998 to July 1999. *Journal of Food Protection,* **65**: 79–87.

Motes, M.L., DePaola, A., Cook, D.W., Veazey, J.E., Hunsucker, J.C., Garthright, W.E., Blodgett, R.J. & Chirtel, S.J. 1998. Influence of water temperature and salinity on *Vibrio vulnificus* in northern Gulf and Atlantic Coast oysters (*Crassostrea virginica*). *Applied and Environmental Microbiology,* **64**: 1459–1465.

Tamplin, M.L. 1994. The seasonal occurrence of *Vibrio vulnificus* in shellfish, seawater, and sediment in United States coastal waters. Final report to Salstonstall-Kennedy Grant Program, US Department of Commerce.

# Appendix E.

# FACSIMILE OF FDA MEMORANDUM

Editor's note: This appendix reproduces an internal memorandum provided to the risk assessment drafting group to assist their work. It has been scanned in from the original hard copy and converted to text using OCR software. The text has received cosmetic attention, but has not otherwise been edited, so it does not conform to the overall style of the rest of the publication.

---

| | |
|---|---|
| To: | Philip C. Spiller<br>Director, Office of Seafood (HFS-400) |
| From: | Karl C. Klontz<br>Medical Officer (HFS-728) |
| Subject: | Estimated number of persons at increased risk for *Vibrio vulnificus* septicemia |
| Date | November 21, 1997 |

Per your request, I have reviewed the 12 November 1997 letter from the Center for Science in the Public Interest (CSPI) in which estimates are provided of the number of persons believed to be at increased risk for acquiring *Vibrio vulnificus* septicemia. Because the estimates in the letter differ from those derived previously by CFSAN, I used this opportunity to reassess FDA's estimates of the number of persons in the U.S. I think could reasonably be considered at increased risk for *Vibrio vulnificus* septicemia.

For each disease, I have provided the reason why persons having the disease are believed to be at increased risk for acquiring *V. vulnificus* septicemia. Because in some instances it is difficult to derive a single number of persons at risk, for some diseases I provide a range, composed of a "low-end" estimate and a "high-end" estimate.

**Diabetes**

The rationale for including diabetics as being at increased risk for acquiring *V. vulnificus* septicemia is a study done in Florida during the 1980s [1] that showed that the risk of infection with *V. vulnificus* was 4.5 times higher among diabetics than among nondiabetics. Acknowledging this, and taking into consideration that, to my knowledge, reports of *V. vulnificus* septicemia occurring among persons with non-insulin-dependent diabetes are very rare, I incorporated the estimated 1,000,000 insulin-dependent diabetics in the U.S. as being at risk. The CSPI number of 16 million clearly includes diabetics who may be on oral therapy or simply on diet/exercise therapy, and the literature does not suggest

*V. vulnificus* septicemia occurs among these persons. Therefore, since there is no documentation that non-insulin-dependents are at increased risk for acquiring *V. vulnificus* septicemia, I have not constructed a range of estimates but provide the single estimate of 1 million persons.

**Alcoholic liver disease**

Alcoholic liver disease is known to be a risk factor for acquiring *V. vulnificus* septicemia. Alcoholic cirrhosis is discovered in 1.6 to 9.9 percent of all necropsies in the U.S. [2]. In 1990, there were approximately 185,000,000 persons over the age of 18 years in the U.S. In my original estimate, I used a value of 2% to estimate the number of adults with alcoholic cirrhosis, thus arriving at a number of 4 million persons. The reason I used a percentage approaching the lower end (i.e., 2%) of the stated range was because I was not certain of the degree to which autopsied individuals truly represent the general population.

Given that there is a range in the estimated proportion of the population that has alcoholic cirrhosis, for the revised estimate I used the upper and lower bounds of the range, yielding an estimates of 2,960,000 (low-end estimate) to 18,315,000 (high-end estimate) persons at increased risk of acquiring *V. vulnificus* septicemia as a result of having alcoholic cirrhosis.

CSPI's estimate is based on "problem drinkers." Like many diseases, alcoholic liver disease represents a spectrum, from mild to severe (cirrhosis). It may be that a proportion of "problem drinkers" are at increased risk for acquiring *V. vulnificus* septicemia prior to getting cirrhosis, but I do not know how to estimate this number. Accordingly, I based the estimate on a clearly defined diagnosis (i.e., cirrhosis) for which I could find population prevalence values in the peer-reviewed medical literature.

**Gastric acidity**

This is one of the "weaker" risk factors for acquiring *V. vulnificus* septicemia. Low gastric acidity clearly is a risk factor for acquiring cholera and some of the other non-cholera vibrios that cause gastroenteritis, but to my knowledge, low gastric acidity has not been established as a risk factor for acquiring *V. vulnificus* septicemia; in fact, in one study [3], use of antacids or cimetidine was shown not to be a risk factor. Nevertheless, there are about 72,000 adults in the U.S. who have had a part or all of their stomach removed (as part of their treatment for gastric cancer) [4], and I have included this estimate into the total.

**Cancer**

The role that cancer plays in placing one at increased risk for acquiring *V. vulnificus* septicemia presumably stems from the interaction of the malignancy itself on a person's immune system or from the effects of chemo- or radiation therapy on the body's immune system. Consequently, in my original estimate of the number of persons at increased risk for acquiring *V. vulnificus* septicemia, I used the number of deaths that occur each year from cancer (i.e., 526,000). Clearly, it is this group of persons who are most debilitated from cancer. It is reasonable to assume that there are cancer patients with disease severe enough to reduce their immune function but who do not die; these individuals would also be at increased risk for acquiring *V. vulnificus* septicemia. Thus, as a revised estimate, I have multiplied my original estimate by a factor of five, thus arriving at a figure of 2,630,000 persons. This figure approximates the number of persons believed to be at increased risk for foodborne disease as cited in a recent report by the Council for Agricultural Science and Technology [5].

In contrast, CSPI indicated a number of 7.4 million cancer patients, citing as a reference for the figure a telephone call to the American Cancer Society. My opinion is that this number is inappropriately large for the purposes of estimating who is truly at increased risk for acquiring *V. vulnificus* septicemia as a result of cancer-associated immune suppression.

**Hepatitis**

As many as 0.2% - 1% of adults in the U.S. show evidence of being chronically infected with hepatitis B virus by virtue of being chronic HBsAg carriers [6]. In addition, surveys of the seroprevalence of antibodies to hepatitis C virus indicate that between 0.2% to 0.6% of volunteer blood donors in the U.S. are infected with hepatitis C virus [6]. Persons chronically infected with either hepatitis B virus or hepatitis C virus often develop cirrhosis of the liver. Thus, based on a U.S. population of 185 million adults, there are an estimated 370,000 - 1,850,000 Americans with chronic hepatitis B virus infection, and 370,000 - 1,110,000 with chronic hepatitis C virus infection.

Persons with chronic hepatitis B virus or hepatitis C virus infection represent a new group added to FDA's previous estimate. The previous estimates inadvertently omitted this group of persons.

**Kidney disease**

CSPI presents a separate category for persons with kidney diseases, estimating this population to consist of 3.5 million persons. The dearth of reported cases of *V. vulnificus* septicemia in the peer-reviewed medical literature suggests that the incidence of infection in this group is extremely low. Nevertheless, one group of persons with kidney disease would be expected to be at increased risk of acquiring *V. vulnificus* septicemia as a result of decreased immune function: those with end stage renal disease. During 1990 in the U.S., approximately 200,000 persons were treated for end stage renal disease [7].

A number of persons with kidney diseases would not be expected to be at increased risk of acquiring *V. vulnificus* septicemia because their disease may not be sufficiently severe to cause decreased immune function. Examples of such persons would be individuals with nephrolithiasis (kidney stones) or microhematuria or mild proteinuria associated with low-gradenephropathies. Additionally, a number of persons with kidney disease that might be severe enough to place them at increased risk for acquiring *V. vulnificus* septicemia would already be included in groups such as those with insulin-dependent diabetes mellitus or cancer. On the other hand, persons whose kidney disease may be a result of autoimmune, rheumatologic, or idiopathic disorders (such as systemic lupus erythematosis or antigen-antibody diseases involving the glomerulus) are included below in a category entitled "conditions associated with decreased immunity."

**Gastritis and duodenitis**

I assume CSPI included these disorders because of the possible decrease in gastric acidity that may be present (particularly for gastritis, but not duodenitis). However, as discussed above in the section on gastric acidity, although low gastric acidity clearly is a risk factor for acquiring cholera and some of the other non-cholera vibrios that cause gastroenteritis, to my knowledge, it has not been established as a risk factor for *vulnificus* septicemia. In fact, in one study [3], use of antacids or cimetidine was shown not to be a risk factor. Thus, I think incorporating the 3.4 million people with gastritis or duodenitis is not reasonable.

**Hemochromatosis**

The estimate FDA used for the number of persons with hemochromatosis was twice as large as that cited by CSPI: FDA used an estimate of 2 million persons, whereas CSPI's estimate was 1 million. We believe the 2 million figure is appropriate, as it factors in persons who may be heterozygous for the condition.

**Conditions Associated with Decreased Immunity**

*AIDS*

CSPI cites a figure of 200,000 to represent persons with AIDS. We believe it may be more appropriate to use a figure of 1 million, which represents a recent estimate of the number of persons in the U.S. infected with HIV [8].

*Persons Receiving Systemic Corticosteroids*

1. **Asthma**. About 5% of the U.S. population has asthma [9]. It is estimated that less than 1% of patients with asthma are dependent on chronic oral steroid therapy [10]. Based on this latter estimate, if one assumes 0.5% as the number of asthmatics who require chronic oral corticosteroid therapy, there are an estimated 47,500 adult asthmatics (195 million persons in U.S. $\geq$ 15 years old $\times$ 0.05 $\times$ 0.005) with impaired immune function due to long-term use of systemic corticosteroid therapy.

2. **Rheumatoid Arthritis**. The prevalence of rheumatoid arthritis is approximately one percent of the population [11], or 1.9 million adults. A study of the use of prednisone by rheumatologists in northern California to treat patients with rheumatoid arthritis indicated that corticosteroids were used in 54% of patient-years (a patient-year is amount of time equivalent to a single patient receiving treatment for one complete year) [12]. Based on this study and the prevalence of rheumatoid arthritis, there are an estimated 950,000 (1.9 million $\times$ 0.54) adults with rheumatoid arthritis in the U.S. treated with corticosteroids.

3. **Psoriatic arthritis**. In the U.S., approximately 1 million persons are affected with psoriasis, and an estimated 7 percent of person with psoriasis experience psoriatic arthritis [13]. Therefore, there are approximately 70,000 persons with psoriatic arthritis, many of whom are treated with systemic corticosteroids.

4. **Systemic lupus erythematosis (SLE).** The prevalence of SLE is estimated to be between 4 and 250 cases per 100,000 population [14], or, at the most, 463,000 persons.

5. **Polymylagia rheumatica (PMR).** The incidence of PMR in the U.S. is estimated to be 53 cases per 100,000 population over the age of 50 years [15]. Therefore, an estimated 34,000 cases of PMR occur every year in the U.S.

6. **Giant cell arteritis (GCA).** The incidence of GCA in the U.S. is estimated to be 12 cases per 100,000 population over the age of 50 years [15]. Therefore, an estimated 7,500 cases of GCA occur every year in the U.S.

**Transplant recipients.** Transplant recipients are at increased risk for acquiring *V. vulnificus* septicemia as a result of taking immunosuppressive medications to prevent organ rejection. There are approximately 110,000 persons living in the U.S. with organ transplants (5).

In summary, using a range approach, the numbers above add up to a "low end" estimate of 11,914,000 and a "high end" estimate of 29,859,000 persons. This contrasts with CSPI's total estimate of 60 million.

Karl C. Klontz, M.D., M.P.H.

**References**

1. Desenclos JCA et al. The risk of *Vibrio* illness in the Florida raw oyster eating population, 1981-1988. American Journal of Epidemiol., 1991; 134:290-297.

2. Boyer TD. Cirrhosis of the liver. In: Cecil Textbook of Medicine. 19th ed. Wyngaarden JE, Smith LH, Bennett JC (eds.) W.B. Saunders, Philadelphia, 1992.

3. Tacket CO et al. Clinical features and an epidemiological study of *Vibrio vulnificus* infections. *Journal of Infectious Diseases* 1984; 149:558-561.

4. Mayer RJ. Neoplasms of the esophagus and stomach. In: Harrison's Principles of Internal Medicine. 13th edition. Isselbacher KJ, Braunwald E, Wilson JD, Martin JB, Fauci AS,

Kasper DL (eds). McGraw-Hill, Inc. New York. 1994.

5. Council for Agricultural Science and Technology. Foodborne Pathogens: Risks and Consequences. Task Force Report No. 122, September 1994.

6. Hsu HH et al. Acute viral hepatitis. In: Principles and Practice of Infectious Diseases. Mandell, Douglas, Bennett (eds). 4th edition. Churchhill Livingstone, New York. 1995.

7. Appel GB. End stage renal disease. In: Cecil Textbook of Medicine. Bennett JC and Plum F (editors), 20th edition. W.B. Saunders, Philadelphia, 1996.

8. Centers for Disease Control and Prevention. 1991 USPHS/IDSA guidelines for the prevention of opportunistic infections in persons infected with human immunodeficiency virus. *MMWR* 1997; 46 (No. RR-12), page 1.

9. McFadden ER. Asthma. In: Harrison's Principles of Internal Medicine. 13th edition. Isselbacher KH, Braunwald E, Wilson JD, Marrtin JB, Fauci AS, Kasper DL (eds). McGraw-Hill, Inc. New York. 1994, page 1167.

10. Barnes PJ, Chung KF. Difficult asthma. Cause for concern. *British Medical Journal* 1989; 299:695-698.

11. Lipsky PE. Rheumatoid arthritis. In: Harrison's Principles of Internal Medicine. 13th edition. Isselbacher KH, Braunwald E, Wilson JD, Martin JB, Fauci AS, Kasper DL (eds). McGraw-Hill, Inc. New York. 1994, page 1648.

12. Criswell LA, Redfearn WJ. Variation among rheumatologists in the use of prednisone and second-line agents for the treatment of rheumatoid arthritis. *Arthritis and Rheumatism* 194; 37:476-480.

13. Ramsay DL, Hurley JJ. Papulosquamous eruptions and exfoliative dermatitis. In: Dermatology. 2nd edition. Moschella SL, Hurley HJ (eds). W.B. Saunders Co. Philadelphia 1985.

14. Schul PH. Systemic lupus erythematosis. In: Cecil Textbook of Medicine. Bennett JC and Plum F (editors), 20th edition. W.B. Saunders, Philadelphia, 1996.

15. Healy LA. Polymyalgia rheumatica and giant cell arteritis. In: Arthritis and Allied Conditions. McCarty DJ, Koopman WJ, (eds). Lea & Febiger, Philadelphia, 1993.

## FAO/WHO MICROBIOLOGICAL RISK ASSESSMENT SERIES

1 Risk assessments of *Salmonella* in eggs and broiler chickens: Interpretative Summary, 2002

2 Risk assessments of *Salmonella* in eggs and broiler chickens, 2002

3 Hazard characterization for pathogens in food and water: Guidelines, 2003

4 Risk assessment of *Listeria monocytogenes* in ready-to-eat foods: Interpretative Summary, 2004

5 Risk assessment of *Listeria monocytogenes* in ready-to-eat foods: Technical Report, 2004

6 *Enterobacter sakazakii* and microorganisms in powdered infant formula: Meeting Report, 2004

7 Exposure assessment of microbiological hazards in food: Guidelines, 2005

8 Risk assessment of *Vibrio vulnificus* in raw oysters: Interpretative Summary and Technical Report, 2005

9 Risk assessment of choleragenic *Vibrio cholerae* 01 and 0139 in warm water shrimp in international trade: Interpretative Summary and Technical Report, 2005